Navigating Long-Term Care
A Reflective Workbook for Nurses

By Sylvia Abbeyquaye, Ph.D. MPA RN

NAVIGATING LONG-TERM CARE WORKBOOK

Copyright © 2023 by Sylvia Abbeyquaye

All rights reserved. No part of this book may be used, reproduced, or stored in a retrieval system or transmitted, in any form or by any means, including mechanical, electronic, photocopy, recording, scanning and methods not invented or in everyday use at the time of this publication, without the prior written permission of the publisher. The use of short quotations or occasional page copying for personal or group study is permitted andencouraged. Permission will be granted upon request.

Publisher
NSD Publishing
www.nsdxpert.com

First Edition
ISBN-13: **979-8-9850972-3-8** - Ebook
ISBN-13: **979-8-9850972-4-5** - Paperback
ISBN-13: **979-8-9850972-5-2** - Hardback

Printed in the
United States of America and United Kingdom

Produced by
Vike Springs Publishing Ltd.
www.vikesprings.com

For bookings and speaking engagements, contact:
nsdxpert@gmail.com
Sylvia's books are available at special discounts when purchased in bulk for training, promotion or as donations for educational and training purposes.

Limit of Liability/Disclaimer of Warranty

This publication is designed to provide accurate and authoritative information regarding the subject matter covered. It is sold with the understanding that the publisher and author are not engaged in rendering medical or clinical advice, and the author makes no representations or warranties with respect to the completeness of the contents of this work. Case studies used in this book are fictitious and solely for educational purposes, and the names of persons or organizations used do not exist. Neither the publisher nor the author shall be liable for damages arising here from. The fact that an organization or website is referred to in this work as a citation and/or a potential source of further information does not mean that the author or the publisher endorses the information that the organization or website may provide or recommendations it may make. Due to the ever-changing information on the web, Internet websites and URLs listed in this work may have changed or been removed. All trademarks or names referenced in this book are the property of their respective owners, and the publisher and author are not associated with any product or vendor mentioned.

PREFACE

This reflective workbook accompanies my new training manual, *"Navigating Long-Term Care: A Practical Approach for Nurses."* Having worked for 20+ years in long-term care settings, I can attest that putting together content and activities for training in long-term care settings can be daunting. Facility nurse educators are pulled to do everything except teach. Therefore, the time to research, prepare, and deliver engaging training sessions is limited. As a result, they resort to presenting quick ad-hoc "re-education" materials on pertinent compliance-related issues. Unfortunately, these pieces of training are ineffective since staff have grown accustomed to them and sign without barely reading the information presented, usually on a clipboard.

Furthermore, the rare in-person training and orientation of new hires are a nightmare since staff often have to sit through boring videos and topics. Orienting new nurses to a facility is a crucial opportunity to foster relationships and help them develop a sense of belonging. It also helps with staff retention and reduces turnover.

It is worth noting that nurses appreciate engaging, interactive training that fosters their professional growth. However, considering the current staffing shortages, it is more urgent than ever before to be creative and adopt a new way of training nurses in long-term care settings.

This book, **"Navigating Long-term Care: A Reflective Workbook for Nurses,"** and its training manual, Navigating Long-term Care: A Practical Approach for Nurses, seeks to bridge these training gaps and enhance quality care delivery.

This 14-chapter workbook sets the stage for active learning and presents engaging individual exercises and group activities. The book uses the nursing process framework to foster critical thinking while learning long-term care procedures. Furthermore, each chapter provides poems, quotes, and questions for self-reflection, allowing the trainee to journal their experiences with the chapter activities and exercises. These reflective activities will help nurses be more mindful on the job and of their self-care to minimize stress. Lastly, the book highlights clinical skills competencies that staff may complete at training.

I encourage trainees to accept this learning approach and allow themselves to grow as long-term care nurses. I suggest a copy of the workbook be given annually to staff during retreats. Also, it can be used as a tool for re-education, where specific chapters are assigned when deficient practice(s) are observed. Finally, this workbook will revamp nursing orientations and improve staff retention and quality care delivery.

Happy reading!

DEDICATION

This workbook is dedicated to all long-term care nurses who care for our population's most vulnerable. But know that your work has gone unnoticed. I commend you for your hard work, tenacity, and resilience. *Keep up the excellent work!*

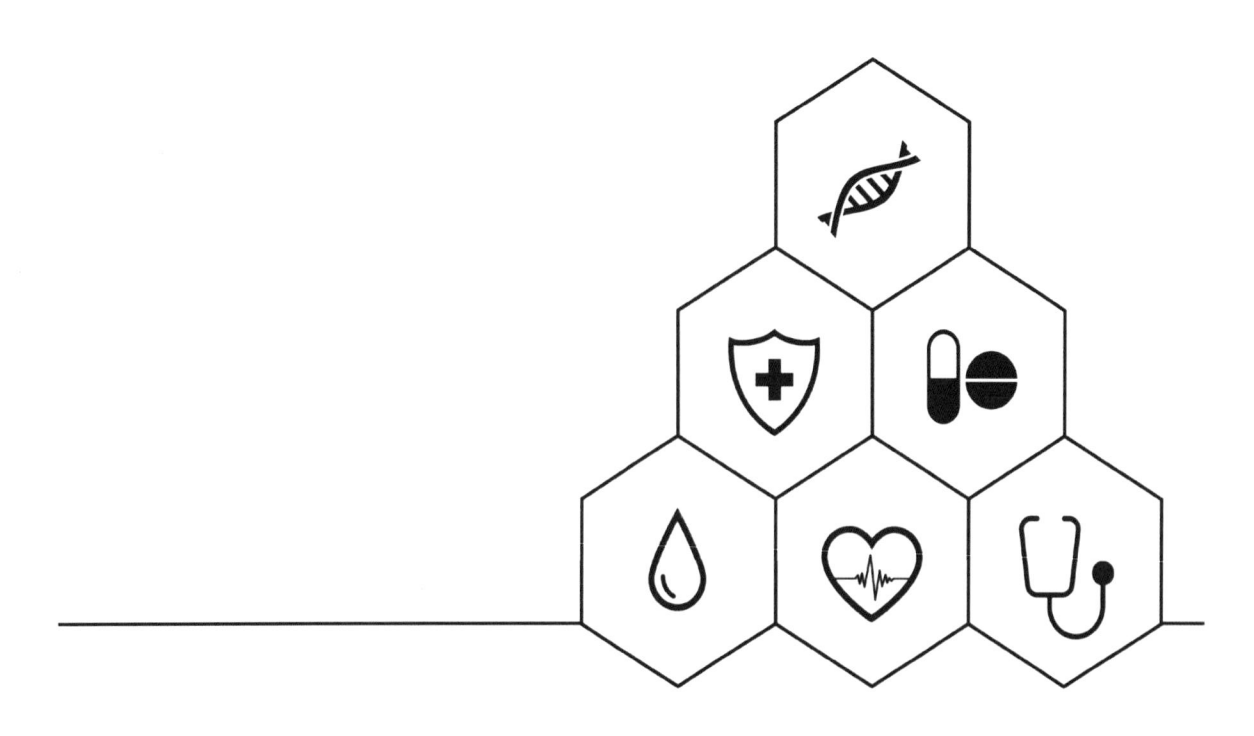

ABOUT THE AUTHOR

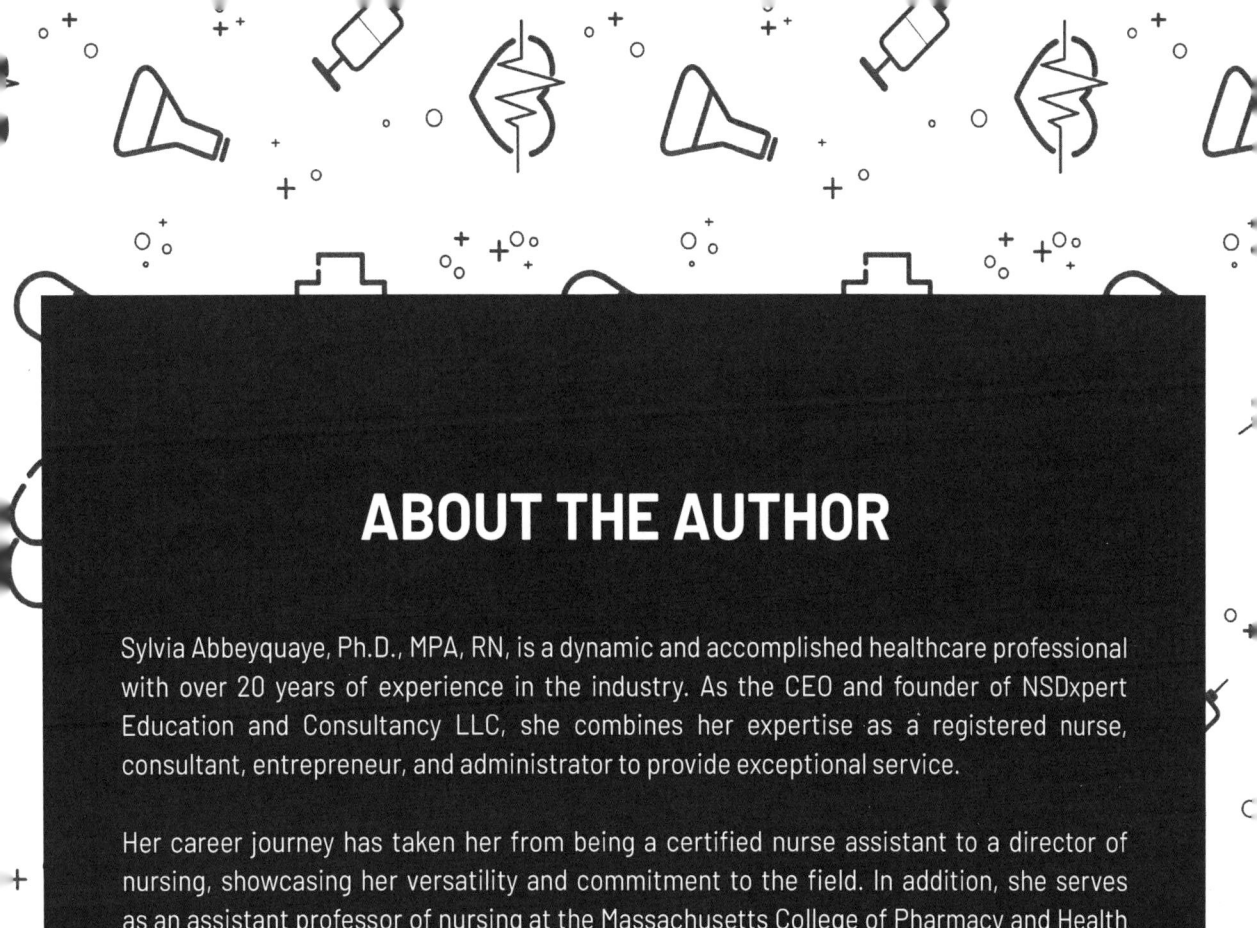

Sylvia Abbeyquaye, Ph.D., MPA, RN, is a dynamic and accomplished healthcare professional with over 20 years of experience in the industry. As the CEO and founder of NSDxpert Education and Consultancy LLC, she combines her expertise as a registered nurse, consultant, entrepreneur, and administrator to provide exceptional service.

Her career journey has taken her from being a certified nurse assistant to a director of nursing, showcasing her versatility and commitment to the field. In addition, she serves as an assistant professor of nursing at the Massachusetts College of Pharmacy and Health Sciences University and as an adjunct professor at the College of Our Lady of the Elms and Endicott College.

She holds a Bachelor of Science in Biochemistry from the University of Science and Technology in Kumasi, Ghana, and a Master's in Public Administration from Clark University in Worcester, Massachusetts. She also earned a Bachelor of Science in Nursing and a Ph.D. in Nursing from the University of Massachusetts, Amherst.

Her passion for healthcare extends to teaching, mentoring new nurses, and advocating for long-term care staff development and retention. Her creation of the NurseLTC app further demonstrates her dedication to the industry. With her vast experience and drive, Dr. Abbeyquaye is an asset to the healthcare community.

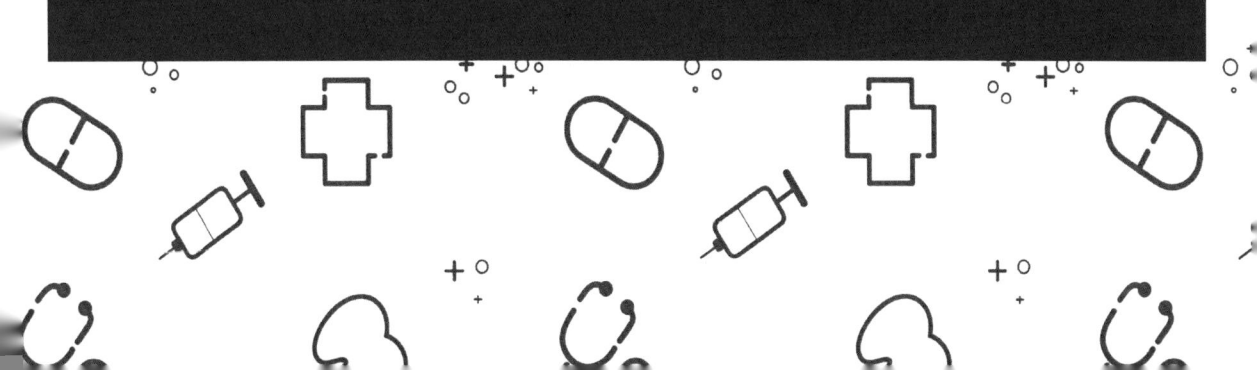

TABLE OF CONTENTS

CHAPTER 1	INTRODUCTION	1
CHAPTER 2	ABOUT YOUR FACILITY	5
CHAPTER 3	ORGANIZATIONAL STRUCTURE	21
CHAPTER 4	YOUR WORK AS A LONG-TERM CARE NURSE	49
CHAPTER 5	CUSTOMER SERVICE	67
CHAPTER 6	COMMUNICATION	77
CHAPTER 7	THE RESIDENT HEALTH RECORD	91
CHAPTER 8	INFECTION CONTROL	101
CHAPTER 9	MEDICATION ADMINISTRATION	115
CHAPTER 10	TREATMENT ADMINISTRATION	127
CHAPTER 11	CLINICAL WORK PROCESSES	135
CHAPTER 12	RESIDENT CARE DELIVERY PROCESS	147
CHAPTER 13	NURSING ASSESSMENTS	165
CHAPTER 14	INCIDENT REPORTING PROCESSES	177

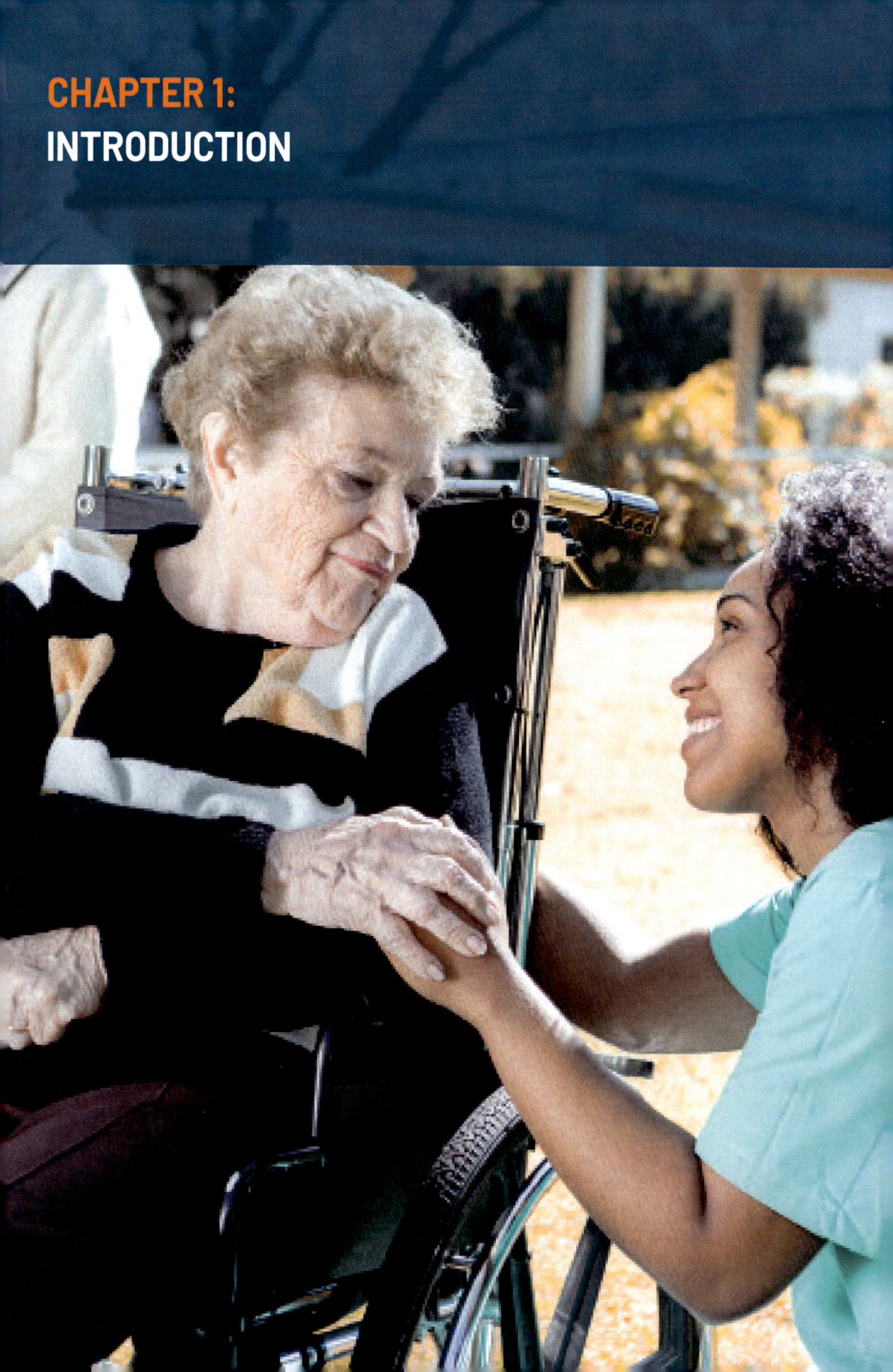

CHAPTER 1:
INTRODUCTION

> "They may forget your name, but they will never forget how you made them feel."
>
> **Maya Angelou**

Following the completion of these exercises, you will be able to:
1. Explain what long-term care nursing practice entails.
2. Explain the concepts of the nursing process model.
3. Apply the nursing process concepts in problem-solving.

Exercise 1

You have been asked to give a speech to a graduating nursing class about what long-term care practice entails. Write what you would include in your address.

Group Activity #1

You have been asked to train a new graduate nurse in long-term care about the nursing process model in care delivery. Develop a teaching plan to:

1. Explain the concepts of the model below:

Assessment → Diagnosis → Planning → Implementation → Evaluation

_____
_____
_____
_____
_____
_____
_____
_____

2. Apply the above concepts to solve an identified issue in your unit. *(You may review Chapter 1 of the training manual to assist you with this exercise).*

_____
_____
_____
_____
_____
_____
_____
_____
_____
_____
_____

CHAPTER 2:
ABOUT THE FACILITY

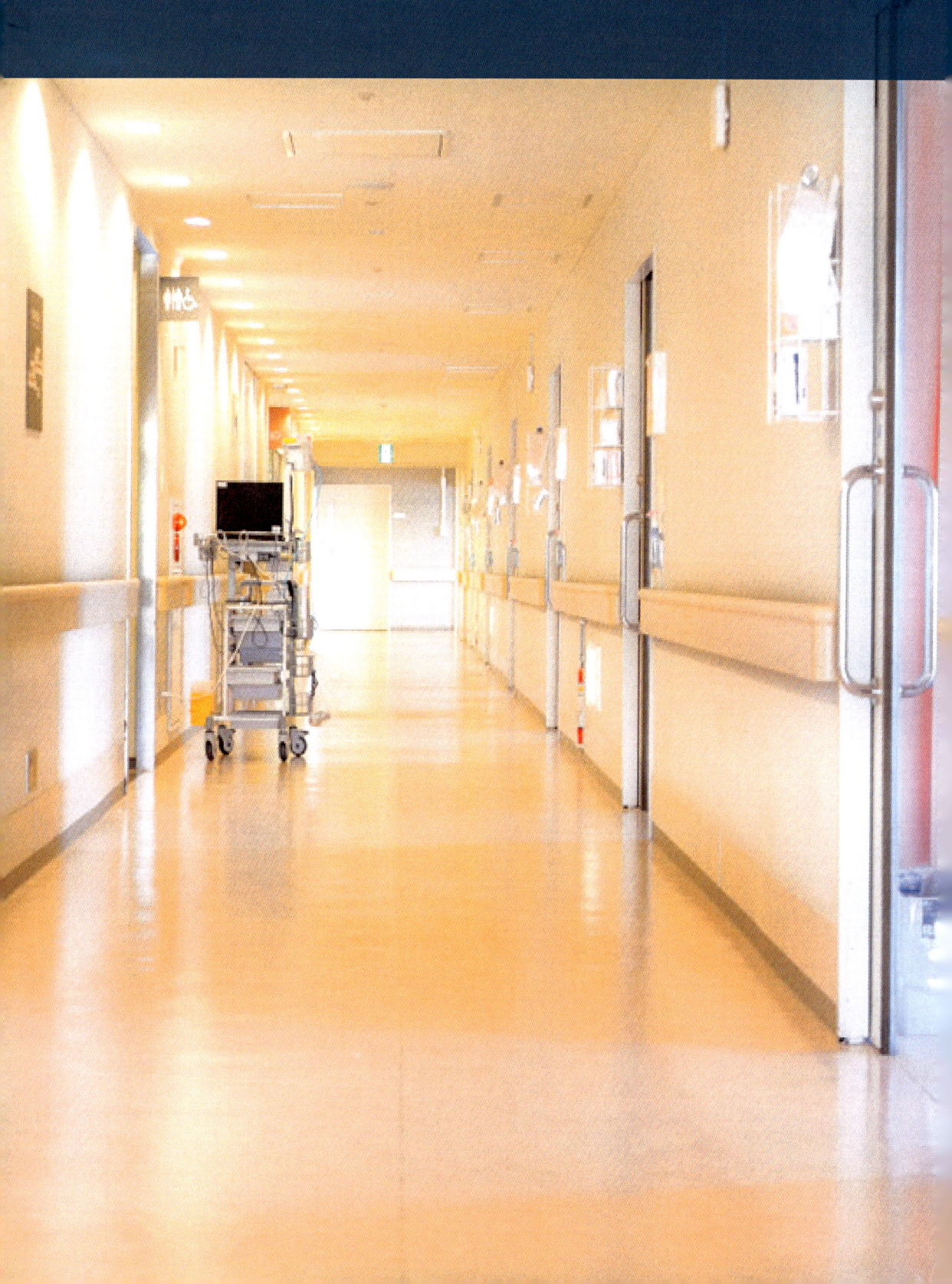

"Your workplace is someone's home. Help make it feel comfortable."

Following the completion of these exercises, you will be able to:
1. Analyze a facility's core mission, vision, and nursing philosophy, and apply them to practice.
2. Analyze the CMS quality star ratings for a long-term care facility and their impact on resident care.
3. Locate vital areas and other resources within an LTC facility to enhance nurses' workflow.
4. Manage staffing issues in a long-term care unit.

Review Chapter 2 of the training manual, *"Navigating Long Term Care: A Practical Approach for Nurses"*, and then attempt the following exercises:

The Characteristics of a Facility

📖 Exercise 1
Analyze your organization's mission and comment on how it may impact your practice as an LTC nurse.

_____
_____
_____
_____
_____
_____
_____
_____
_____
_____
_____
_____
_____
_____
_____
_____
_____

Exercise 2

Analyze your organization's vision and comment on how it may impact your practice as an LTC nurse.

___

Exercise 3

In a few sentences, write how you can help advance the mission and vision of your organization.

Exercise 4

Give an example of an instance where your practice as a nurse aligned with your organization's mission and vision.

Nursing Philosophy/ Theory

Exercise 5

What is the nursing philosophy or theory followed by your organization?

Exercise 6

Explain how the theory or philosophy guides your organization's clinical practices.

Exercise 7

If your organization does not have a guiding nursing philosophy or theory, use a selected theory, e.g., Orem's theory of self-care, and outline how that may guide your practice as a nurse within your organization.

Facility Layout

Group Activity #1

Take a tour of your facility or engage in a scavenger hunt. Then indicate where you will locate the following:

1. Code cart(s)
2. Automated External Defibrillator (AED)
3. Eye wash stations
4. Dirty utility room
5. Specimen refrigerator
6. Mailroom
7. Nursing supply stock room
8. General supplies stock room
9. Nursing Policy and Procedure manual
10. Material Safety Data Sheet (MSDS) Manual
11. Laboratory requisition book
12. Resident appointment book
13. Linen closet
14. Oxygen storage room
15. Office of the Director of Nursing
16. Unit manager's office
17. Unit kitchenette
18. Training/computer room
19. Staff break room
20. Payroll office

Exercise 8

Does knowing the location of the key resources listed above impact your workflow as a nurse in a long-term care facility? Explain.

_____
_____
_____
_____
_____
_____
_____
_____
_____
_____
_____
_____

Staffing

Case Study Review

Refer to the case study, "Staff Shortage at Akwaaba Skilled Nursing Facility" on page 15 of your training manual and answer the following questions:

A. How should Rose Doe (RN) have assessed the situation?

_____
_____
_____
_____
_____
_____
_____
_____
_____
_____

B. What are some questions she should have asked to understand the situation at hand better?

_____
_____
_____
_____
_____
_____
_____
_____
_____
_____

C. What plan could she have developed to mitigate this situation?

D. What interventions could she have put in place?

E. Reflect on the case presented and evaluate what could be considered in preventing a future occurrence of such situations.

___

Facility Quality Indicators and CMS Quality Star Ratings
Group Activity #2

As a group, discuss your experiences with the DPH survey process and what lessons you took away from the process.

Look up your facility's quality star ratings report and answer the following questions:

Exercise 9
How many deficiency tags do you have, and how severe are they?

___

Exercise 10
Reflect and write briefly about how these tags may influence resident care.

Exercise 11
What is the current plan(s) of correction in place at your facility?

Exercise 12

If you are a new hire, how do you intend to help adhere to the correction plan? Describe.

_____
_____
_____
_____
_____
_____
_____
_____
_____
_____

Exercise 13

If you are currently an employee, describe what you are doing to help adhere to the plan of correction. Give a specific example(s).

_____
_____
_____
_____
_____
_____
_____
_____
_____
_____

Exercise 14

Suppose you were given your facility as an inheritance. List two things you would do differently to enhance the quality of care for the residents at the facility.

Case Study Review

Refer to your training manual's case study on page 20 and answer the following questions:

A. What is the nurse's role in maintaining compliance at Akwaaba Skilled Nursing Center?

_____

_____

_____

_____

_____

_____

_____

_____

_____

B. Based on the case scenario, how did the survey affect the work process for the nurses at Akwaaba Skilled Nursing Center?

_____

_____

_____

_____

_____

_____

_____

_____

_____

_____

C. As a new hire at Akwaaba Skilled Nursing Center, do you think knowing the facility's survey results would affect your practice? Explain.

Author's Reflection

"Though my efforts seem to go unnoticed, I strive to be the best nurse I can be. I look at the frail and vulnerable people I have been assigned to work for, and I am encouraged and strengthened to do my very best to achieve excellence, often with limited resources. Yet, I do this diligently and sometimes with pain because I know I will be there one day and want my nurse to care for me just as I have."

Self-Reflective Exercise

Stop for a few minutes and reflect by asking yourself these questions.

1. How can I make this facility a home for my residents and myself?
2. What can I do to help build a more substantial working community?
3. What should I do to integrate myself fully into the culture of my facility?
4. Will I bring my loved one to be taken care of at this facility?
5. What can I do to help improve the quality of care at this facility?

My Journal

CHAPTER 3:
ORGANIZATIONAL STRUCTURE

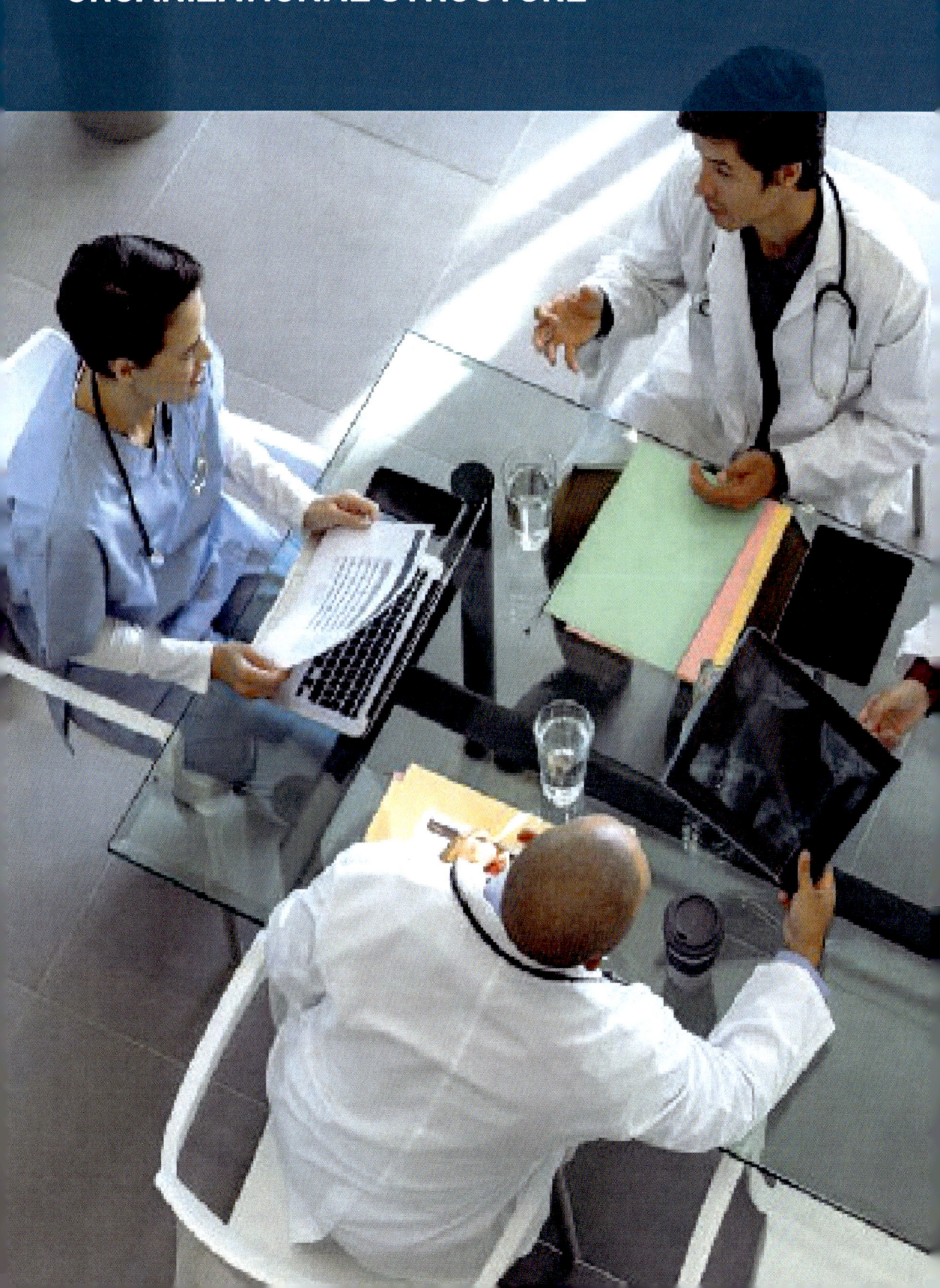

> "He who thinks he is leading and has no one following him is only taking a walk."
>
> **African proverb.**

Following the completion of these exercises, you will be able to:
1. Describe crucial roles within a long-term care nursing department and their impact on practice.
2. Interpret the nursing department's organizational hierarchy.
3. Interpret a nursing job description and the responsibilities of an LPN/RN in a long-term care facility.
4. Interpret the seven essential roles of a long-term care nurse.
5. State your commitment against incivility and bullying in the workplace.
6. Reflect on your role as a long-term care nurse.

Review Chapter 3 of the training manual, "Navigating Long Term Care: A Practical Approach for Nurses", and then attempt the following exercises:

Key Roles within the Nursing Department

Exercise 1

Name the Executive Director (ED) and state their organizational role.

_____
_____
_____
_____
_____
_____
_____
_____
_____
_____
_____
_____
_____
_____

Exercise 2

Describe how the ED's role impacts your practice as a nurse within the facility.

_____

_____

_____

_____

_____

_____

_____

_____

_____

_____

Exercise 3

Name the Director of Nursing (DON) and state their organizational role.

_____

_____

_____

_____

_____

_____

_____

_____

_____

_____

Exercise 4

Describe how the DON's role impacts your practice as a nurse within the facility.

___

Exercise 5

Using your training manual's sample organizational chart on **page 27**, identify your role and interpret its chain of command. (The people you may report to). *If you have an organizational chart, you may use that instead.*

Exercise 6

Review and interpret your facility's job description. Then, in your own words, describe your responsibilities as an LPN or RN.

_____

_____

_____

_____

_____

_____

_____

_____

_____

_____

(New hires may be asked to sign their job descriptions after this exercise)

The Nurse as a Leader

Exercise 7

In your own words, describe who a leader is.

_____

_____

_____

_____

_____

_____

_____

_____

_____

_____

Exercise 8

Interpret the image below:

_____
_____
_____
_____
_____
_____
_____
_____
_____
_____
_____
_____

Take a few minutes to reflect on your previous responses, then answer the following questions:

Exercise 9

Do you consider yourself a leader? Explain.

_____
_____
_____
_____
_____
_____
_____
_____
_____
_____
_____
_____
_____

📖 Exercise 10

How easily can you ask the CNAs assigned to work with you to complete their task efficiently?

📖 Exercise 11

How do you handle a situation when a certified nurse assistant refuses to do a task you assigned?

Exercise 12

What is your style of leadership? Give an example from your practice.

Exercise 13

What will you do as the nurse (LPN or RN) on duty if a fire starts on your unit during the 11-7 shift?

The Nurse as a Manager

Case Study Review #1

Read the case study, "Whose Job Is It", on page 32 of your training manual, and answer the questions.

A. Who is a nurse manager?

_____
_____
_____
_____
_____
_____
_____
_____
_____
_____
_____
_____

B. Did Nurse Petunia make the right decision?

_____
_____
_____
_____
_____
_____
_____
_____
_____
_____
_____
_____

C. What, if anything, should have been done differently in the case study?

D. Whose role is it to ensure the medication cart is well stocked and medications are reordered?

The Nurse, as a Caregiver

📖 Exercise 14

What does it mean to be considered a caregiver?

_____

_____

_____

_____

_____

_____

_____

_____

_____

📖 Exercise 15

List three characteristics you would want to have as a nurse caregiver.

_____

_____

_____

_____

_____

_____

_____

_____

_____

_____

_____

Exercise 16

In your role as a caregiver, list three things that have been your most significant challenges.

___

Case Study Review #2

Refer to the case study, "The Role of the Nurse," on page 33 of your manual and provide the answers to questions A and B below

A. ___

B._____

_____
_____
_____
_____
_____
_____
_____
_____
_____
_____
_____
_____
_____
_____
_____
_____
_____
_____
_____
_____

The Nurse as an Advocate

This poem was found among the possessions of an elderly lady who died in the geriatric ward of a hospital. No information is available concerning her, who she was, or when she died.

It was reprinted from the "Assessment and Alternatives Help Guide" prepared by the Colorado Foundation for Medical Care.

Take a moment to reflect on the poem "See Me" and answer the questions.

Poem: See Me

What do you see, nurses, what do you see?
What are you thinking when you look at me —
A crabby old woman, not very wise,
Uncertain of habit, with far-away eyes,
Who dribbles her food and makes no reply,
When you say in a loud voice — "I do wish you'd try."

Who seems not to notice the things that you do,
And forever is losing a stocking or shoe,
Who, unresisting or not, lets you do as you will,
With bathing and feeding, the long day to fill.
Is that what you're thinking? Is that what you see?
Then open your eyes, nurse, you're looking at ME...
I'll tell you who I am as I sit here so still.
As I rise at your bidding, as I eat at your will.

I'm a small child of ten with a father and mother,
Brothers and sisters, who love one another,
A young girl of sixteen with wings on her feet.
Dreaming that soon now a lover she'll meet.
A bride soon at twenty — my heart gives a leap,
Remembering the vows that I promised to keep.
At twenty-five now, I have young of my own,
Who needs me to build a secure, happy home.
A woman of thirty, my young now grow fast,
Bound to each other with ties that should last;
At forty, my young sons have grown and are gone,
But my man's beside me to see I don't mourn;
At fifty, once more babies play 'round my knee,
Again, we know children, my loved one, and me.

Dark days are upon me; my husband is dead,
I look at the future; I shudder with dread,
For my young are all rearing young of their own,
And I think of the years and the love that I've known;
I'm an old woman now, and nature is cruel —

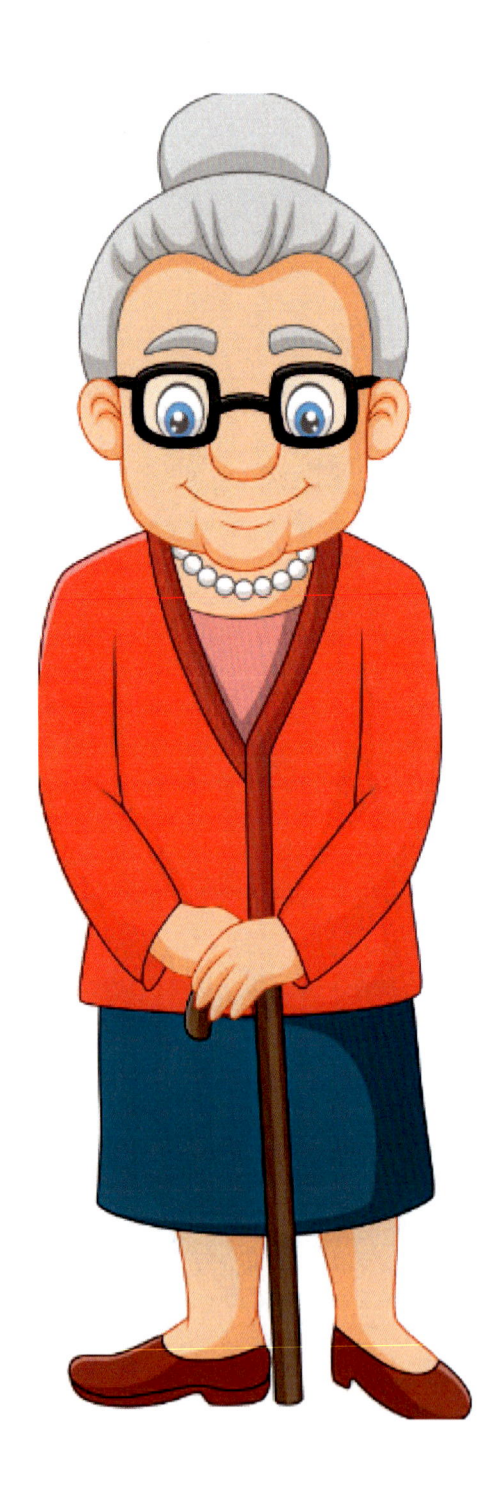

'Tis her jest to make old age look like a fool.
The body is crumbled, grace and vigor depart,
There is now a stone where once I had a heart,
But inside this old carcass, a young girl still dwells,
And now and again, my battered heart swells.

I remember the joys; I remember the pain,
And I'm loving and living life over again,
I think of the years, all too few — gone too fast,
And accept the stark fact that nothing can last —
So, I open your eyes, nurses, open and see,
Not a crabby old woman; look closer, nurses — see ME! - **Unknown Author**

Group Activity #1

Form a group with your peers, review and discuss the poem above, and answer the following questions:

1. What is the author trying to tell the nurses caring for her?

_____

_____

_____

_____

_____

_____

_____

_____

_____

_____

_____

_____

_____

_____

2. As an advocate for your residents, what could you do for residents like the poem's author?

Case Study Review #3

Read the case study, "The Nurse's Role in Advocacy", on page 35 of your training manual and answer the questions below.

A. Is there an advocacy role for the nurse in this case?

B. What should Nurse Albert do to handle this case?

C. Who should Nurse Albert advocate for in this case?

Nurse as a Mentor

"The key to being a good mentor is to help people become more of who they already are, not to make them more like you " — Suze Orman.

Exercise 17

a) Do you have a nurse mentor?

_____
_____
_____
_____
_____
_____
_____
_____
_____
_____

b) If yes, how have you benefited from that relationship?

_____
_____
_____
_____
_____
_____
_____
_____
_____
_____

c) If not, then what has been the barrier to having a mentor?

Exercise 18

What desirable attributes would you want in a mentor?

Exercise 19

As a mentor, give an example where you demonstrated any of the desirable attributes mentioned earlier toward your mentee.

_____
_____
_____
_____
_____
_____
_____
_____
_____
_____

Group Activity #2

As a group, brainstorm and discuss some strategies you may use to find a mentor and develop a mutually beneficial relationship.

Case Study Review #4

Refer to the case study on mentorship on page 35 of the training manual and answer the questions below.

A. Who is a nurse mentor?

_____
_____
_____
_____
_____
_____
_____
_____

B. How would you assess the case?

C. Do you agree with Nurse Bullyson's assessment of the current generation of nurses? Explain.

D. As a coworker on the unit, what support will you provide Nurse Abena, if any?

The Nurse as a Companion

Case Study Review #5

Read the case study, "Can Companionship be Delegated", page 37 of the training manual, and answer the questions below.

A. What do you make of the case scenario?

B. Did the nurse make the right decisions in this case? Why?

C. Do you think the nurse provided companionship to Mr. Williamson in this case? Explain.

Self-Reflective Exercise

Close your eyes and look within yourself. Who do you see? A bully? A victim? A survivor, or neither?

Stop for a few minutes and reflect by asking yourself these questions.

Am I kind to my coworkers and residents?

How can I be an effective mentor to others?

Do I fulfill all the roles of a long-term care nurse?

Am I tolerant of the new nurse on a unit?

As a caregiver, do I have empathy for the residents?

What can I do to be a better version of myself?

Are my coworkers eager to work after me?

Exercise 20

Write a commitment to yourself about addressing bullying and incivility and how you want to be treated at the workplace.

My Journal

CHAPTER 4:

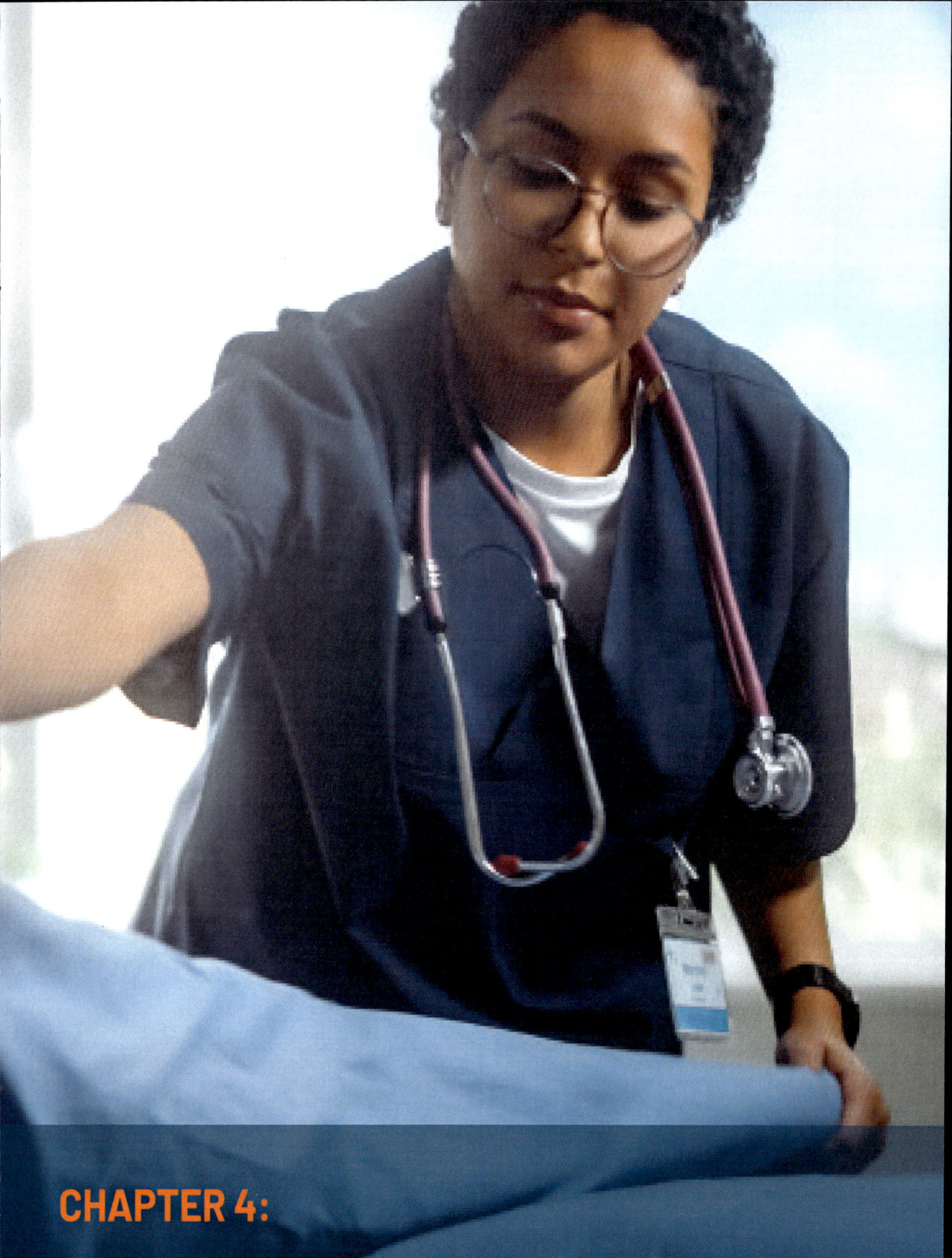

YOUR WORK AS A LONG-TERM CARE NURSE

"A person who does no hard work will never know the value of rest."
- African Proverb

Following the completion of these exercises, you will be able to:
1. Categorize and prioritize the daily long-term care nurse tasks.
2. Analyze the three types of nurse tasks in long-term care settings.
3. Create a task plan to enhance work efficiency.
4. Discuss disciplinary actions in long-term care.
5. Distinguish between team members and team players.
6. Identify barriers to teamwork.
7. Describe the essential elements of teamwork.
8. Use technology for time management.

Review Chapter 4 of the training manual, *"Navigating Long Term Care: A Practical Approach for Nurses"*, and then attempt the following exercises:

Daily Nurse Tasks- Clinical / Operational / Organizational

Exercise 1
For new graduate nurses, only
Review the sample shift checklist in Appendix A of your training manual and categorize the listed tasks as clinical, operational, or organizational.

Clinical Tasks	Operational Tasks	Organizational Tasks

Exercise 2

a. Reflect on the assigned duties and responsibilities and outline a realistic plan to complete tasks efficiently.

_____

b. Outline how each task category from exercise 1 may benefit the resident.

_____

Exercise 3

For all other facility nurses

a. Outline, in order of priority, your typical workday tasks. Then, compare it to the sample shift checklist in Appendix A of your training manual and identify tasks that may be new to you or the least prioritized. Explain

b. Categorize the new or least prioritized tasks as clinical, operational, or organizational.

Clinical Tasks	Operational Tasks	Organizational Tasks

c. Comment on what you found.

_____
_____
_____
_____
_____
_____
_____
_____
_____
_____
_____
_____
_____
_____

📖 Exercise 4

Using the work process template in Appendix A of the training manual, develop a realistic plan to share with a new graduate nurse to complete all their tasks efficiently and effectively.

Group Activity #1

You are a skilled nursing facility nurse who notices the workload is impossible. In fact, since the COVID-19 pandemic, no one has wanted to work, and the facility is increasingly using agency staff. You and your peers wonder how to provide quality care to all residents without creating workarounds. Also, you are increasingly worried you may make significant errors due to the heavy workload and violate your professional code of conduct and license. Furthermore, you feel angry and hate the job you once loved. You want to fix a broken system. As a nurse, what should you do?

A. As a team, outline a realistic plan to present to the Director of Nursing to create your dream workplace.

Disciplinary Action

Case Study Review #1

Read the case study on page 46 and answer the following questions:

A. What is your opinion on this case?

B. Using your facility's disciplinary policy as a guide, do you think the Director of Nursing should have fired Nurse Melly? Explain.

C. Do you think Nurse Melly followed the standards of nursing practice? Explain.

D. What are some factors that could have been influencing Nurse Melly's behavior?

The Nursing Team

"Teamwork begins by building trust. And the only way to do that is to overcome our need for invulnerability."
– Patrick Lencioni.

📖 Exercise 5

Based on the definitions outlined in Chapter 4 of the training manual, are you a team member or a team player? Explain.

_____
_____
_____
_____
_____
_____
_____
_____
_____
_____
_____
_____

📖 Exercise 6

A CNA tells the nurse, "I just come in, do my job, and leave. When there is a call out, I will never stay, so do not bother to call me". If you were the nurse, what would you do?

_____
_____
_____
_____
_____
_____
_____
_____
_____
_____
_____

Exercise 7

What are some barriers that may impede teamwork within a facility?

Case Study Review #2

Refer to the case study, "Teamwork and Discharge Planning," on page 49, and answer the following questions:

A. Discuss the elements of teamwork identified in the case presented.

B. What should have been done differently, if anything?

C. What was the role of the nurse in discharge planning?

D. Assuming Mr. Hillsburg got home and his services were not in place, what could the facility have done to resolve the issue?

Time Management Using the Nursing Process

"You will never find time for anything. If you want time, you must make it"
- Charles Buxton.

Case Study Review #3

Refer to the case study, "Nurse Madeline's Day at Work," on page 52, and answer the questions below.

A. Using the nursing process, outline how nurse Madeline can manage her time during this shift.

B. The case does not outline everything that Nurse Madeline must do. Instead, list other tasks a 7-3 nurse will do in a long-term care facility.

C. Create a task plan for nurse Madeline based on her daily nursing tasks. The plan must outline functions that could be prioritized, delegated, or completed together with her peers.

D. Complete the work process worksheet in Appendix A of the training manual to outline the task plan created.

___

📖 Exercise 8

The NurseLTC ® application uses the nursing process as a time management tool. Download it from the Google Play Store and take a few minutes to review how it works and how to navigate its use in your work process.

The Florence Nightingale Pledge

"I solemnly pledge myself before God and in the presence of this assembly, to pass my life in purity and to practice my profession faithfully. I will abstain from whatever is deleterious and mischievous and will not take or knowingly administer any harmful drug. I will do all in my power to maintain and elevate the standard of my profession. I will hold in confidence all personal matters committed to my keeping and all family affairs coming to my knowledge in the practice of my calling. With loyalty, will I endeavor to aid the physician in his work and devote myself to the welfare of those committed to my care."

Self-Reflection Exercise

Stop for a few minutes and reflect by asking yourself these questions.

1. Am I living up to Florence Nightingale's pledge when caring for my residents?
2. Why did I choose nursing as a career?
3. How do I practice as a long-term care nurse?
4. How do my actions impact resident care delivery?
5. How can I be a solution to the staffing problems my facility is facing?
6. How can I help to improve the quality of care provided at this facility?
7. How can I be the best version of myself?

My Journal

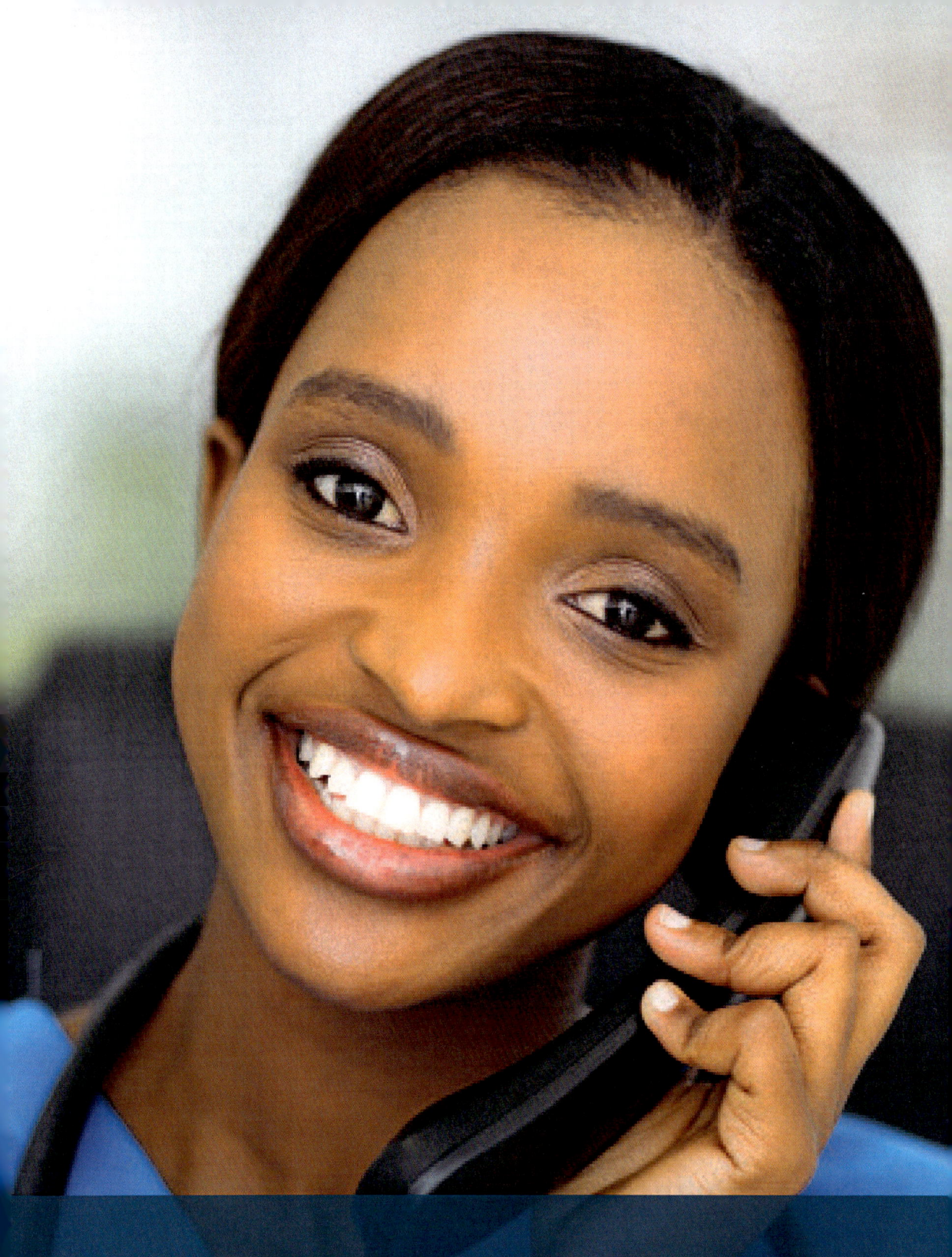

CHAPTER 5:
CUSTOMER SERVICE

> "Your customer doesn't care how much you know until they know how much you care."
>
> **- Damon Richards**

Following the completion of these exercises, you will be able to:

1. Understand the importance of customer service in a long-term care facility.
2. Recognize good customer service practices.
3. Interpret Brownlee's principles of good customer service in care delivery?
4. Handle a dissatisfied customer.
5. Formulate a grievance report.
6. Evaluate customer service practices in care delivery through self-reflection.

Review Chapter 5 of the training manual, "Navigating Long Term Care: *A Practical Approach for Nurses*", and then attempt the following exercises:

The Principles of Customer Service

Exercise 1

Have trainees role-play a phone conversation between a nurse and an angry family member using the script below.

Staff Nurse:
Hello, how may I help you?

Family Member:
WHO AM I SPEAKING TO?

Staff Nurse:
My name is Susan Mingle. I am the nurse on duty.

Family Member:
Fine! Is there a supervisor I can talk to?

Staff Nurse:
Not currently. Who am I talking to, and how may I help you?

Family Member:
I do not understand what you just said. Do you mean there is no supervisor at the facility? Then let me talk to whoever can answer my questions.

Staff Nurse:
I need to know exactly what you are looking for so I can direct you to the person who can help you.

Family Member:
I visited my mother over the weekend, and she told me the nurses do not give her medications. My mother has high blood pressure, and she needs her pills. Nobody knows what they are doing there!

Staff Nurse:
Who is your mother?

Family Member:
Cecelia Perry

Staff Nurse:
And which daughter am I talking to?

Family Member:
Agnes [family member pauses] Agnes Williams

Staff Nurse:
Please hold for a minute.

"The nurse puts the family member on hold and grabs the resident's health record to verify who is listed as the resident's responsible person. After 2 minutes, the nurse returns to the phone".

Staff Nurse:
Hello, Sorry for keeping you waiting. Our records do not list you as a responsible party, and I cannot share any further information with you.

Family Member:
HOW DARE YOU TALK TO ME LIKE THAT! MY SISTER AMY IS THE HCP, BUT SHE IS AWAY ON VACATION, AND YOU MEAN I CANNOT CHECK ON MY MOTHER?

Staff Nurse:
I did not say that. I said that because of HIPAA rules, I could not disclose personal information unless your mother or the health care proxy said it was OK.

Family Member:
THIS PLACE IS A DUMP! I KNEW IT. YOU DO NOT TAKE GOOD CARE OF THE RESIDENTS. MY MOTHER HAS HAD 3 FALLS SINCE SHE CAME HERE. WAIT TILL I CALL THE STATE ON YOU.

Staff Nurse:
You may go ahead. I must go now.

Family Member:
I cannot believe you are so rude. I will report you to your supervisor and get you fired.

Staff Nurse:
OK. bye

"The family member hangs up".

Reflect on the role-play scenario presented above and answer the following questions:

a. Analyze and describe what just happened in this scenario.

b. Did Nurse Susan follow any of David Brownlee's customer service principles?

c. What could have been done differently in this case?

d. Based on the family member's grievances, file a report using your facility's grievance form or the sample in Appendix B of your training manual.

e. Reflect on a similar or unpleasant encounter with a customer at the facility and briefly describe what happened and how you handled it.

___

📄 Case Study Review #1

Refer to the case study, "Customer Service-Family Grievance," and answer the questions below.

A. Did Nurse Amy show good customer service?

___

B. What could she have done differently?

C. What elements of customer service may have been missed in the interaction between Nurse Amy and Mrs. Johnson? Discuss.

D. What is the process of handling a grievance at your facility?

Self-Reflective Exercise

Stop for a few minutes and reflect by asking yourself these questions.

- How do I serve my customers?
- What makes me upset when dealing with an angry customer?
- How can I be assertive with my customers without being rude?
- How does my practice of customer service impact resident care?
- What is my attitude toward our customers?

My Journal

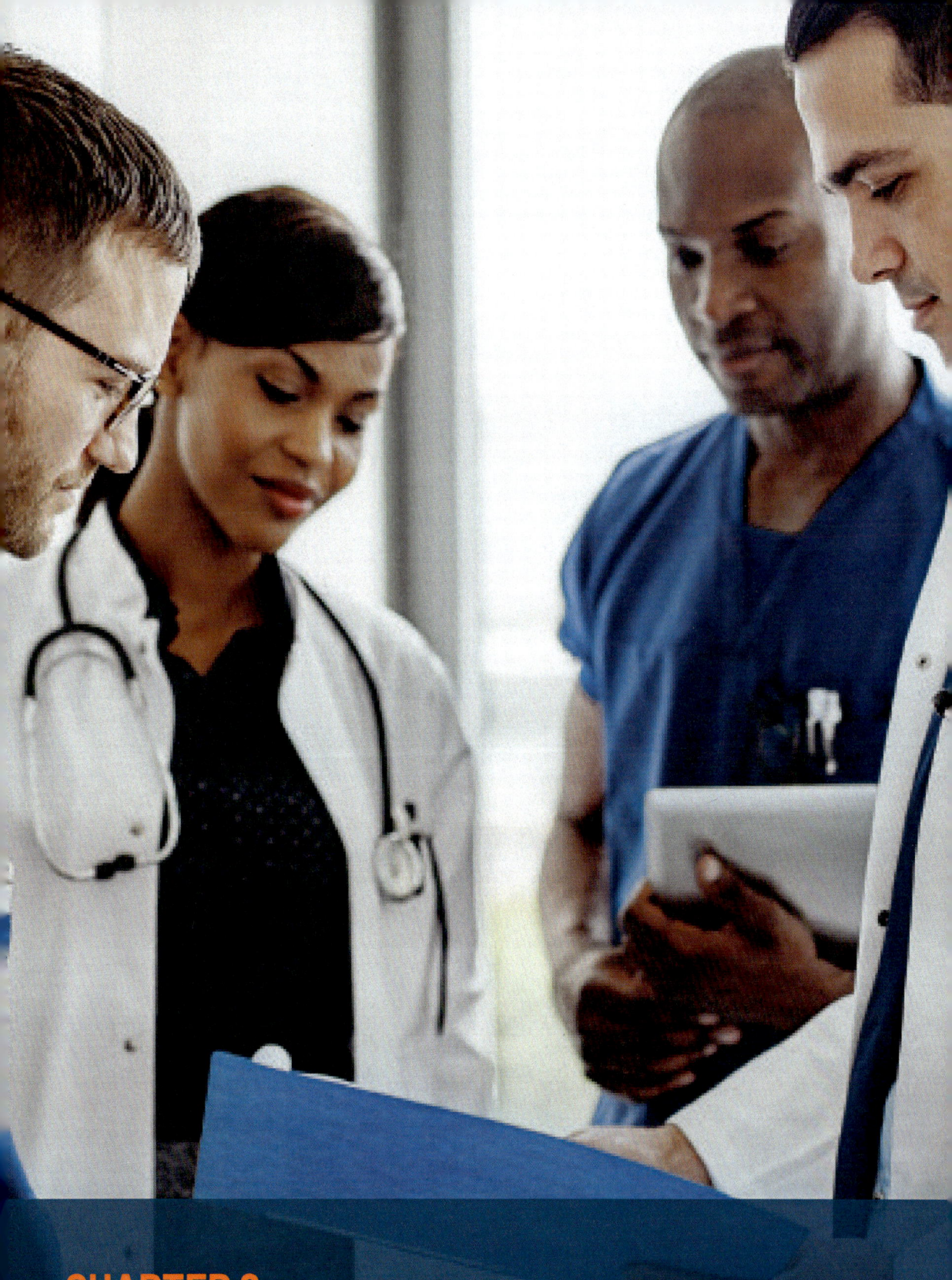

CHAPTER 6:
COMMUNICATION

"Just because the lizard nods its head does not mean it's in agreement."
- African Proverb

Following the completion of these exercises, you will be able to:
1. Recognize the elements of effective communication.
2. Evaluate the elements of effective communication in long-term care delivery.
3. Identify the different modes of communication.
4. Use phone technology effectively to enhance workflow.
5. Complete an SBAR tool for communication during care delivery.
6. Engage in interprofessional communication with the care team.

Review Chapter 6 of the training manual, "Navigating Long Term Care: A Practical Approach for Nurses" and then attempt the following exercises:

The Principles of Effective Communication

Exercise 1

Attend a clinical huddle, care planning, risk management, or discharge planning meeting and answer the questions below.

a. In a few sentences, analyze what you observed at the meeting.

___
___
___
___
___
___
___
___
___
___
___
___
___
___

b. Comment on effective communication at this meeting, highlighting the positive and negative aspects.

Exercise 2

Transfer a call, answer a call, and print a test page out. Describe what you learned in the process.

📖 Exercise 3

Explore each page of your organization's intranet, and in a few sentences, summarize what was communicated to you and other employees.

_____

_____

_____

_____

_____

_____

_____

_____

_____

_____

_____

📖 Exercise 4

Visit your organization's website and summarize what was communicated to you and the public.

_____

_____

_____

_____

_____

_____

_____

_____

_____

_____

Exercise 5

After analyzing the information from the organization's internet and intranet, is their communication effective? Explain

Exercise 6

a. Take a resident's health record and read the social worker's admitting note. What message was relayed to you through that note?

b. Was it new information, and will the message help you provide better care for the resident? Explain

___

Group Activity #1

Have trainees listen to an audio recording of a shift report and take notes. Review and critique for the accuracy of their report notes as a group.

Case Study Review #1

Review the case study below and answer the following questions:

> Mrs. Janice Green is an 80-year-old resident assigned to Nurse Lucy on the 7-3 shift. Nurse Lucy noticed a 6 cm x 8 cm skin tear during her routine rounds on Mrs. Green's right arm. However, due to her advanced dementia, Mrs. Green could not indicate how she sustained the injury. Upon further inquiry, the CNA Eunice said that Mrs. Green has been aggressive with staff lately, especially during her showers, and sometimes it takes two aides to get her ready for bed. The CNA, Eunice, and the staff present denied witnessing any incident that may have caused the skin tear. Nurse Lucy provided first aid to stop the bleeding and called the covering clinician to update them on the resident's status. The clinician then asked Nurse Lucy to do the following:
>
> - Obtain CBC, BMP, and UA C+S in the AM.
> - Wash the wound with NS, apply Bacitracin, and, then cover it with a non-adhesive dressing.
> - Refer for a psychiatric consultation.
>
> The orders were transcribed and followed as directed. Finally, at the end of the shift, the Nurse Lucy documented and reported the incident to the incoming nurse.

1. List all the modes of communication Nurse Lucy may have utilized in this scenario.

2. If you were the nurse, write your report to the incoming nurse.

Before calling the clinician, Nurse Eunice used the SBAR template to communicate effectively. What could she have written? Refer to **pages 71-73** of the training manual.

S. _____

B. _____

A.

R.

# Case Study Review #2

Refer to the case study, *"Communication"*, on page 74 of your manual, and answer the following questions:

A. Using the SBAR communication tool, outline how Nurse Eric should communicate the situation to Dr. Freely and the oncoming nurse in the end-of-shift report.

B. List the different modes of communication that could be used in this case.

C. How would you ensure that communication is effective in such a scenario?

Group Activity #2

Take a tour of the facility's designated photocopy/fax room. Each team member may demonstrate using the fax machine and related features, such as photocopying, document scanning, and e-mail.

Self-Reflective Exercise

Stop for a few minutes and reflect by asking yourself these questions.

How often do I listen to respond?

How often do I listen to understand?

How do I communicate unpleasant news to others?

How does terrible communication affect my work?

How do I communicate with my residents and peers?

What can I do to improve my communication with my peers?

My Journal

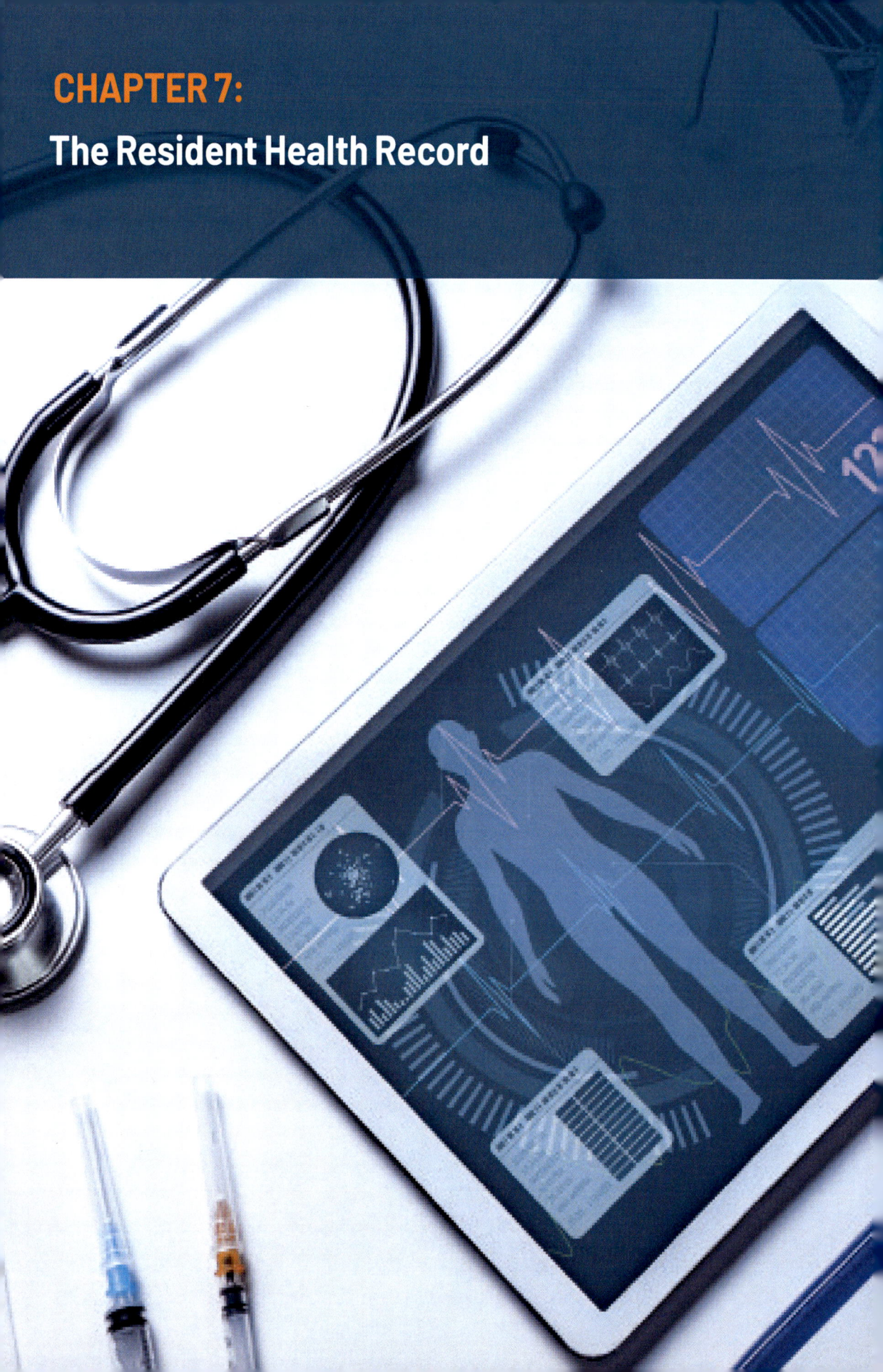

CHAPTER 7:
The Resident Health Record

Good record-keeping improves workflow and enhances efficiency.

Following the completion of these exercises, you will be able to:
1. Locate vital residents' health records needed to enhance quality care delivery.
2. Organize a resident's health record accurately to enhance the nurse's workflow.
3. Describe the role of the nurse in resident health record management.
4. Apply HIPAA guidelines to medical record requests and handling.

Review Chapter 7 of the training manual *"Navigating Long Term Care: A Practical Approach for Nurses"* and then attempt the following exercises.

The Sections of a Resident's Chart

Exercise 1

Navigate a resident's chart and your facility's Electronic Health Record System to find and record the location of the following information:

ITEM	LOCATION(S)
Primary physician's name and address	
Resident's payor source	
MOLST form	
Admission date	
Resident's age	
Healthcare proxy information	
Resident's allergy status	
Admitting diagnosis	
Hospital discharge summary	
Physician orders	
Consent for treatment	
Medication administration record	
Immunization record	
Admission intake assessment form	
Treatment administration record	
Covid-19 status of the resident	
ADL care plan	

ITEM	LOCATION(S)
Psych consult report	
Progress notes (physician, nurses, dietician, therapists)	
Social Worker(s)	
Minimum Data Set (MDS)	
Consent for psychotropic medication	
Fall risk assessment form	
Wound consult report	
Falls care plan	
Preadmission Screening and Resident Review (PASRR)	
Guardianship paperwork	
Incident report	
ADL flow sheet	
Last CBC lab report	
Kardex for CNAs	
Resident's Inventory list	
Brief Interview for Mental Status (BIMS) score	
Previous month's nursing summary	
Annual health and physical report	
Last month's pharmacy recommendation	

Exercise 2

How does the location of these residents' health records impact your practice as a nurse in a long-term care facility?

Exercise 3

What is your role as a long-term care nurse in managing residents' health records?

Exercise 4

Complete a 24-hour chart audit to ensure all new clinician orders are processed and posted on the Medication Administration Record (MAR).

_____

_____

_____

_____

_____

_____

_____

_____

_____

_____

Case Study Review #1

Refer to the case study, "HIPAA and Handling Medical Records", on page 87 of your training manual, and answer the following questions:

a.   Who is a covered entity under HIPAA regulations?

_____

_____

_____

_____

_____

_____

_____

_____

_____

_____

b. Identify if there were HIPAA violations in this case.

c. Did Nurse Petunia act appropriately with Priscilla? Explain.

d. What, if anything, would you have done differently in such a situation?

e. Does Priscilla have the right to discharge her mother from the facility?

Self-Reflective Exercise

Stop for a few minutes and reflect by asking yourself these questions.

Do I return the resident's chart to the rack after using it?

Do I file loose medical reports I find at the nurses' station in the correct place?

Do I take time to review medical records flagged in the residents' charts?

Do I find time to ensure MOLST and consent forms are signed before filing them away?

Do I complete 24-hour chart audits to prevent medication errors?

My Journal

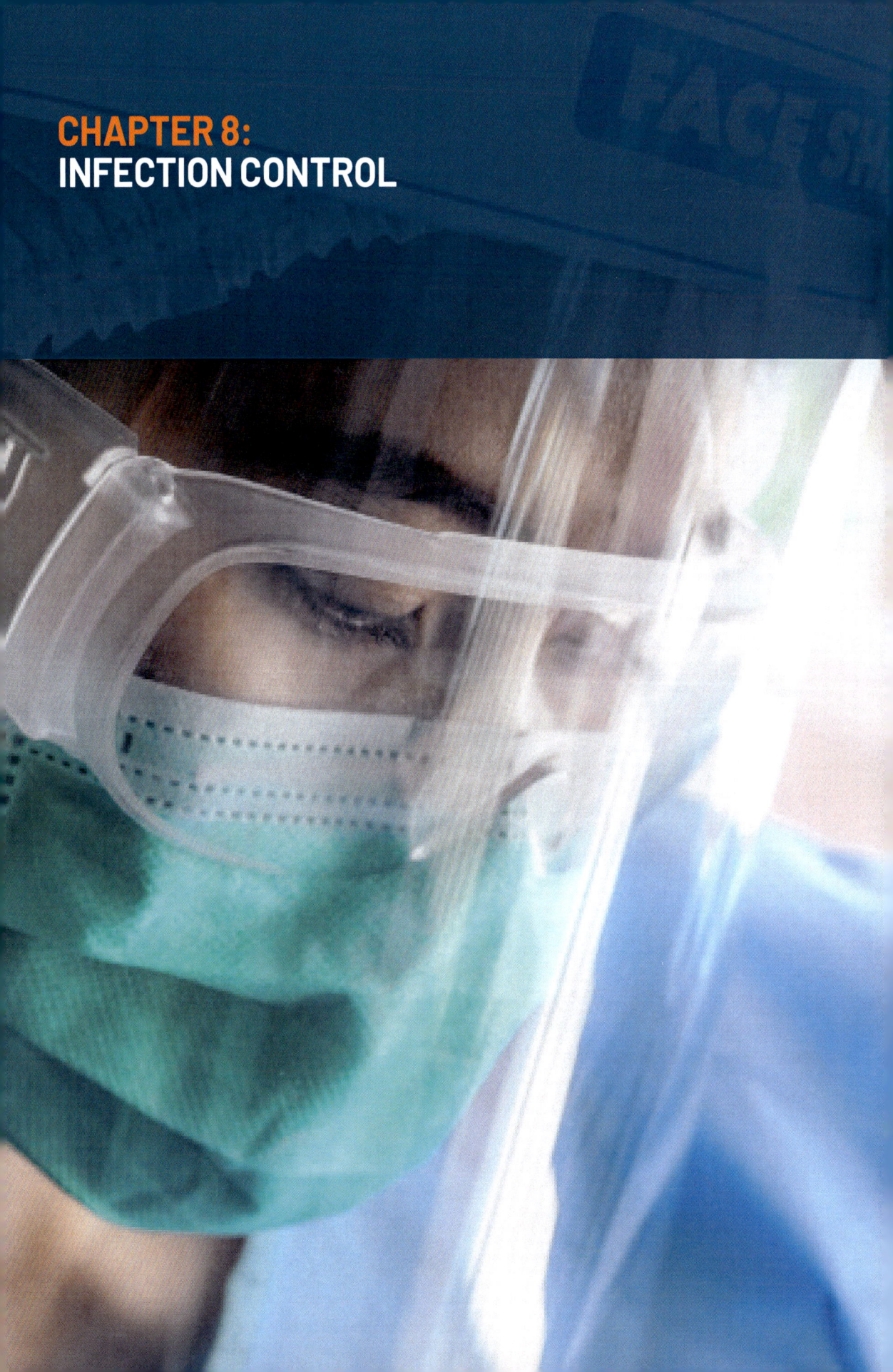

CHAPTER 8:
INFECTION CONTROL

> "Care is an absolute. Prevention is the ideal."
>
> - Christopher Howson

Following the completion of these exercises, you will be able to:
1. Outline a lesson plan? about the chain of infection and infectious disease transmission.
2. Apply infectious disease transmission principles in outbreak prevention and management of COVID-19 and other diseases.
3. Describe the infectious disease management processes used in long-term care.
4. Apply standard precautions in resident care delivery.
5. Describe enhanced barrier precautions.
6. Describe vaccine storage and handling.
7. Demonstrate infection control clinical skills competency.
8. Explain antibiotic stewardship.

Review Chapter 8 of the training manual, "Navigating Long Term Care: A Practical Approach For Nurses", and then attempt the following exercises:

Infectious Disease

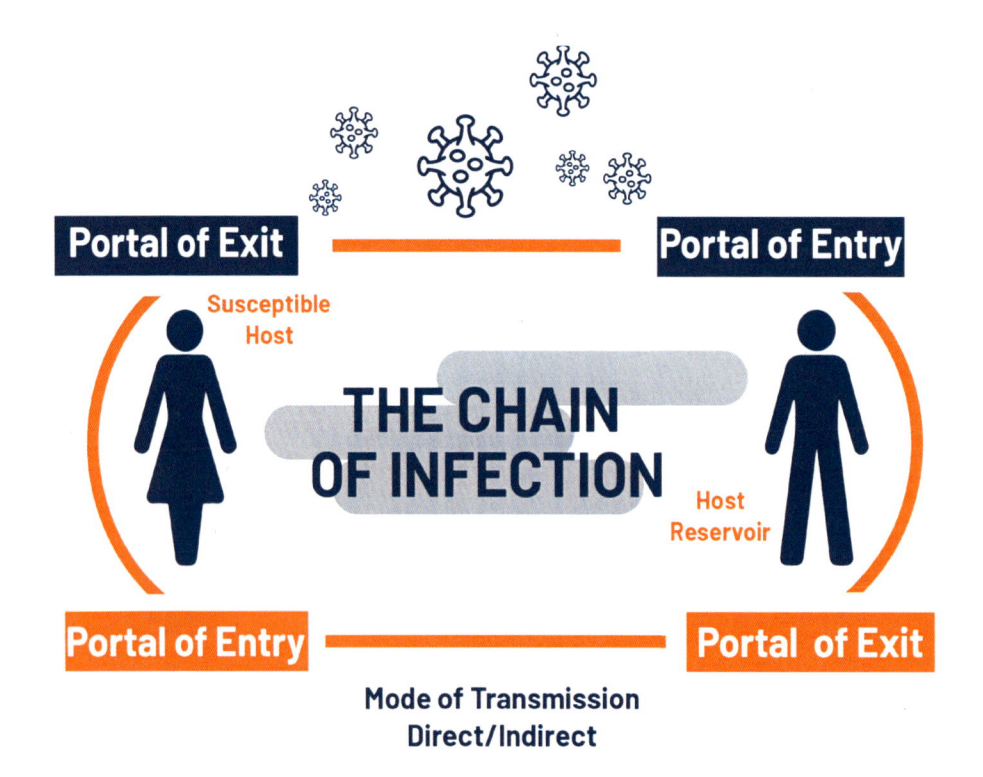

THE CHAIN OF INFECTION

- Portal of Exit
- Portal of Entry
- Susceptible Host
- Host Reservoir
- Portal of Entry
- Portal of Exit
- Mode of Transmission Direct/Indirect

Exercise 1

As part of a QAPI initiative at your facility, you have been asked to lead a team in developing a lesson plan about the chain of infection and infectious disease transmission. Based on Chapter 8 of your training manual, outline the information you would include in your plan.

Standard Precautions

Exercise 2

Take a tour of a nursing unit, and based on your understanding of standard precaution measures, identify instances where standard precautions were not followed and list the infractions below.

Exercise 3
Give two suggestions to improve compliance with standard infection control at your facility.

Clinical Skills Competency

1. **Demonstrate how you would perform hand hygiene.**

    a. Using soap and water

    b. Using alcohol hand sanitizer

2. **Demonstrate how to don and remove Personal Protective Equipment (PPE)**

Exercise 4

The Centers for Disease Control and Prevention (CDC) has updated their guidance on enhanced barrier precautions (EBP) for all healthcare settings, including nursing homes. Review the guidelines at the link below and answer the following questions:

https://www.cdc.gov/hai/pdfs/containment/Letter-Nursing-Home-Staff-508.pdf

A. How are you implementing these guidelines in your practice? Explain.

Exercise 5

You have been asked to precept a new graduate nurse hired on your unit. What will you teach them about the facility's policy on the following:

A. Infectious disease outbreak management (COVID-19, Norovirus, Influenza, and Legionnaires disease)?

_____

_____

_____

_____

_____

_____

_____

_____

_____

_____

B. Vaccine storage and handling?

_____

_____

_____

_____

_____

_____

_____

_____

_____

C. Antibiotic stewardship?

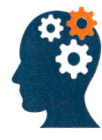

Clinical Skills Competency

- Isolation procedures
- Point of care testing (POCT) and specimen collection
    - COVID-19
    - Flu
    - Blood glucose test
    - Occult blood test (Guaiac)
- Vaccination administration
- Mantoux testing for tuberculosis

Group Activity #2

Pair up with a peer and conduct infection control rounding on a nursing unit. Use the infection control daily walking rounds checklist provided in **Appendix C** of your training manual. Discuss your findings with your peers.

Case Study Review #1

Refer to the case study, "A Gastrointestinal Infection Outbreak in a Skilled Nursing Facility", and answer the questions below:

A. Describe what may be going on at Akwaaba Skilled Nursing Center.

_____
_____
_____
_____
_____
_____
_____
_____
_____
_____

B. What are contact precautions?

_____
_____
_____
_____
_____
_____
_____
_____
_____
_____
_____
_____

C. Why did the MD order contact precaution?

D. What infection control practices should Nurse Amanda educate her nurse aides about?

E. Describe how the outbreak can be managed at the facility.

F. Describe the nurse's role in infection control practices.

Self-Reflective Exercise

Stop for a few minutes and reflect by asking yourself these questions.
1. What infection control measures do I take to keep myself, residents, and staff safe?
2. How often do I observe infection control practices?
3. Do I wipe down the blood pressure cuff in between resident uses?
4. Do I disinfect the medication cart often during med pass?
5. How often do I disinfect the glucometer in between resident uses?

My Journal

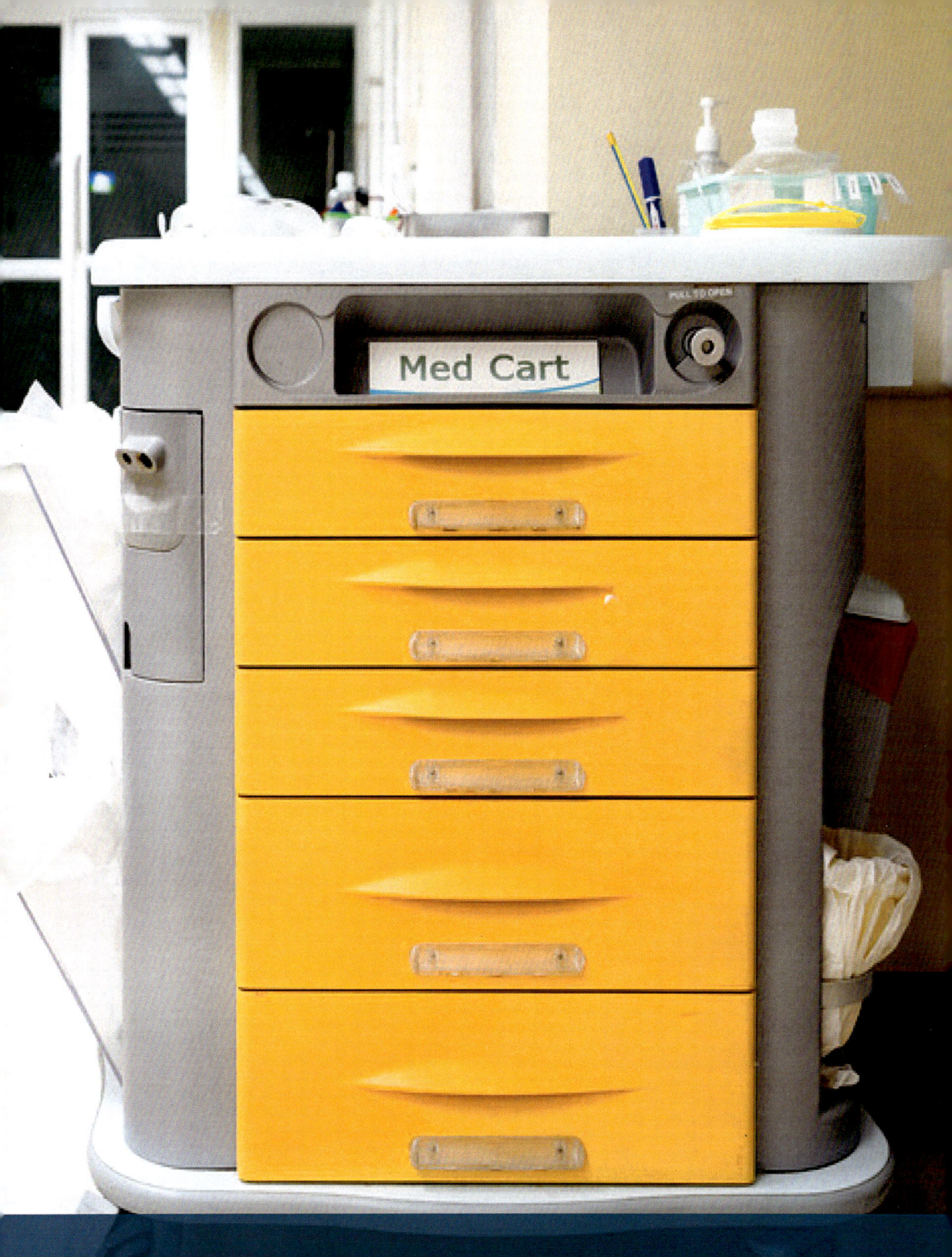

CHAPTER 9:
MEDICATION ADMINISTRATION

"The single greatest impediment to error prevention in the medical industry is that we punish people for making mistakes."

- Lucian Leape

Following the completion of these exercises, you will be able to:
1. Apply concepts of the nursing process in medication administration.
2. Apply the principles of the five rights of medication administration.
3. State the causes of medication errors in long-term care facilities.
4. Outline strategies to prevent medication errors.
5. Review the handling and management of controlled substances in a long-term care facility.
6. Create a teaching plan for managing and administering psychotropic medications.
7. Demonstrate clinical competency in medication administration.
8. Manage a discrepancy in the narcotics count.

Review Chapter 9 of the training manual, "Navigating Long Term Care: A Practical Approach for Nurses" and then attempt the following exercises:

Exercise 1
Describe your process of medication administration, starting with your cart preparation.

Exercise 2
Analyze how the process you described above aligns with the concepts of the nursing process (assessment, diagnosis, planning, implementation, and evaluation)

Exercise 3
In your opinion, what are the causes of medication administration errors in long-term care?

Exercise 4

List at least five strategies you use to prevent medication administration errors.

Group Activity #1

CMS regulates the safe administration of psychotropic medications (antidepressants, mood stabilizers, antipsychotics, anxiolytics, stimulants, and sleep aids). Research and prepare a teaching plan to educate new graduate nurses on these regulations. Include your group's method of evaluating their understanding of the presentation.

___

Case Study Review #1

Refer to the case study, "A Significant Medication Error," on page 131 of your training manual, and answer the questions below:

A. What are the five rights of medication administration?

B. What could have caused this medication error?

Statements obtained during the investigation revealed that Nurse Marigold pre-pours most of her medications and keeps them in the medication cart.

C. Give two reasons why pre-pouring medicine is an unsafe method of medication administration.

D. What is your opinion on terminating Nurse Marigold's employment at the facility?

E. What would you have done differently in this case?

Exercise 5

Describe what you would do as the incoming nurse when a discrepancy is found during a narcotic count at the start of your shift.

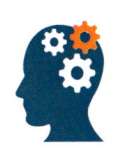

Clinical Skills Activities

Demonstrate competency in administering medications using the following routes:

- Oral route of administration
- Tablets/capsule
- Liquid medication
- Sublingual route of administration
- Rectal route of administration
- Gastrointestinal tube administration
- Nasal route of administration
- Use of dry powdered inhalers
- Metered dose inhalers
- Soft mist inhalers (nebulizers)
- Intravenous (IV) route of administration
- Peripheral
- Midline
- Central line
- Care of Intravenous site and dressing change
- Peripheral cannula IV insertion
- The intramuscular route of administration
- The subcutaneous route of administration
- Intradermal route of administration
- Eardrop administration
- Eyedrop and ointment administration
- Narcotic count

Self-Reflective Exercise

Stop for a few minutes and reflect by asking yourself these questions.

1. Do I keep the medication cart clean and organized?
2. Do I restock the cart when supplies are low?
3. Do I reorder medications from the pharmacy when supplies are low?
4. Do I log the refrigerator's temperature?
5. Do I report any medication errors I did or noted?
6. Do I date all opened insulin vials and other medications?
7. Do I document insulin site rotation?
8. Do I assess blood pressure before administering antihypertensives?
9. Do I check the apical pulse before giving Digoxin®?
10. Do I give all my medications when I'm running out of time?
11. How do I execute my medication pass when no one is looking?

My Journal

CHAPTER 10:
TREATMENT ADMINISTRATION

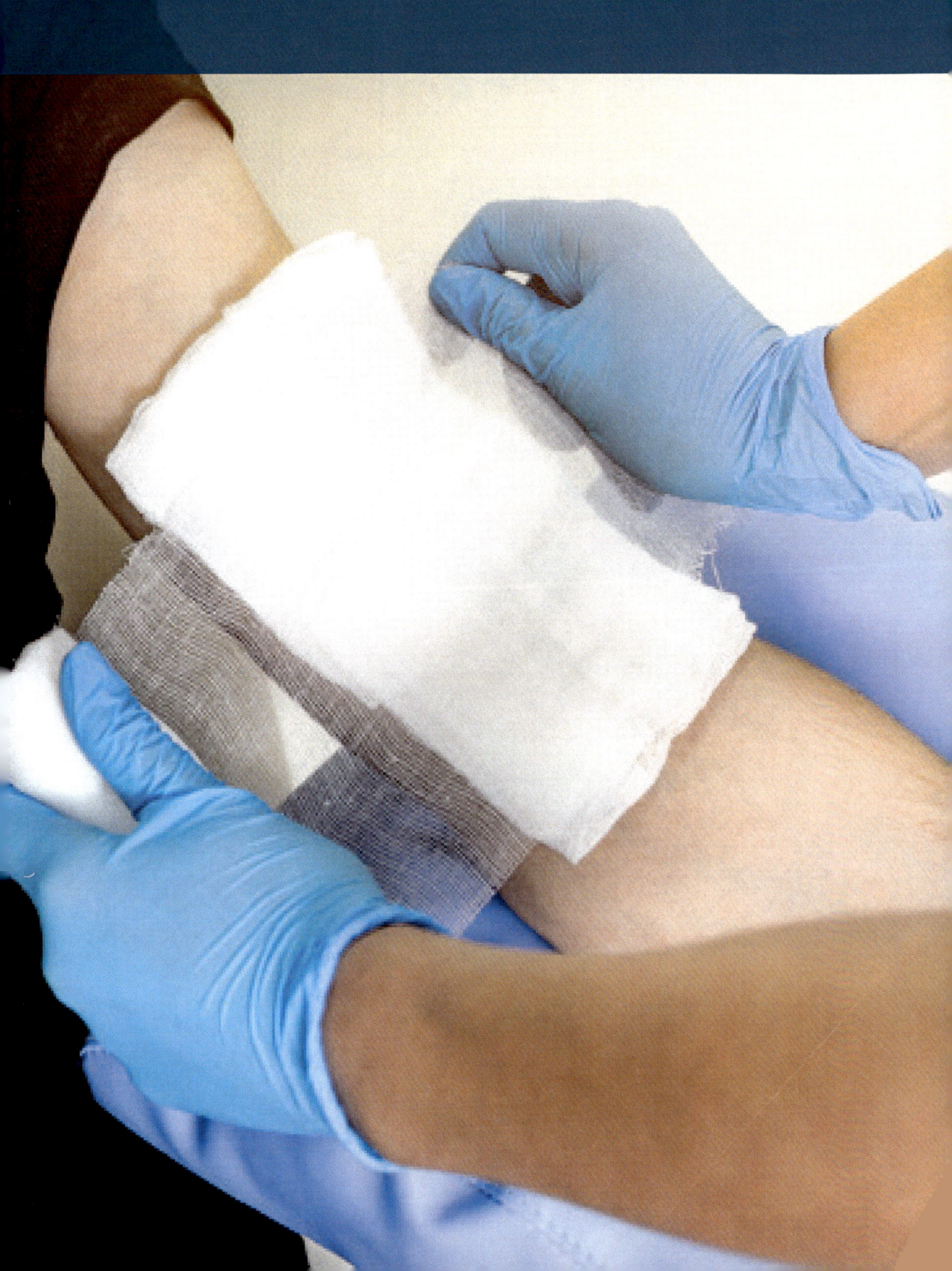

Following the completion of these exercises, you will be able to:
1. Apply the concepts of the nursing process in treatment administration.
2. Demonstrate competency in safe treatment administration.
3. Describe the role of the long-term care nurse in chronic wound management.
4. Demonstrate competency in wound measurement and documentation.
5. Demonstrate competency in specimen collection.

Review Chapter 10 of the training manual *"Navigating Long Term Care: A Practical Approach for Nurses"* and then attempt the following exercises:

The Process of Treatment Administration

Exercise 1
Describe your process of treatment administration, starting with the preparation of the cart.

_____
_____
_____
_____
_____
_____
_____
_____
_____
_____
_____
_____
_____
_____

Exercise 2

Outline how your process described above aligns with the nursing process concepts of assessment, diagnosis, planning, implementation, and evaluation.

Wound Management and the Nurse's Role

Exercise 3

What is your role in the management and prevention of:

a. Pressure ulcers?

b. Vascular ulcers?

c. Diabetic ulcers?

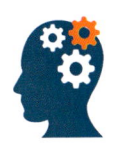

Clinical Skills Competency

Demonstrate competency in the following areas:
- Wound measurement
- Wound dressing changes
- Negative pressure wound therapy
- Wound vac dressings
- Sterile dressing procedure
- Clean dressing procedure
- Foot care
- Diabetic foot care
- Donning and removing thromboembolic deterrent (TED) stockings
- Insertion of an indwelling catheter
- Irrigation of an indwelling catheter
- Care of an indwelling catheter
- Care of a suprapubic catheter
- Suprapubic catheter dressing change
- Measuring post-void residuals using a bladder scanner
- Surgical drain care
- Drain flushing
- Tracheostomy care
- Change of inner cannula
- Tracheostomy suctioning procedure
- Oral suctioning procedure
- Deep suctioning procedure
- Tracheostomy dressing change
- Gastrointestinal (G) tube care
- G-tube dressing change
- Mouth care
- Colostomy care
- Ileostomy care
- Sample collection
  - Urine
  - Clean catch urine
  - Foley catheter collection
  - Stool
  - Nasal swab
- Respiratory equipment use
- Oxygen concentrator
- Oxygen cylinders and change of tubing
- Nebulizers and change of tubing.
- Care of BiPAP/CPAP

Self-Reflective Exercise

Stop for a few minutes and reflect by asking yourself these questions.
1. What do I do when I notice a treatment error (e.g., a missed treatment)?
2. Do I keep the treatment cart stocked and organized?
3. Do I provide detailed documentation after treatment is completed?
4. How do I perform my treatment administration when no one is looking?

My Journal

CHAPTER 11:
CLINICAL WORK PROCESSES

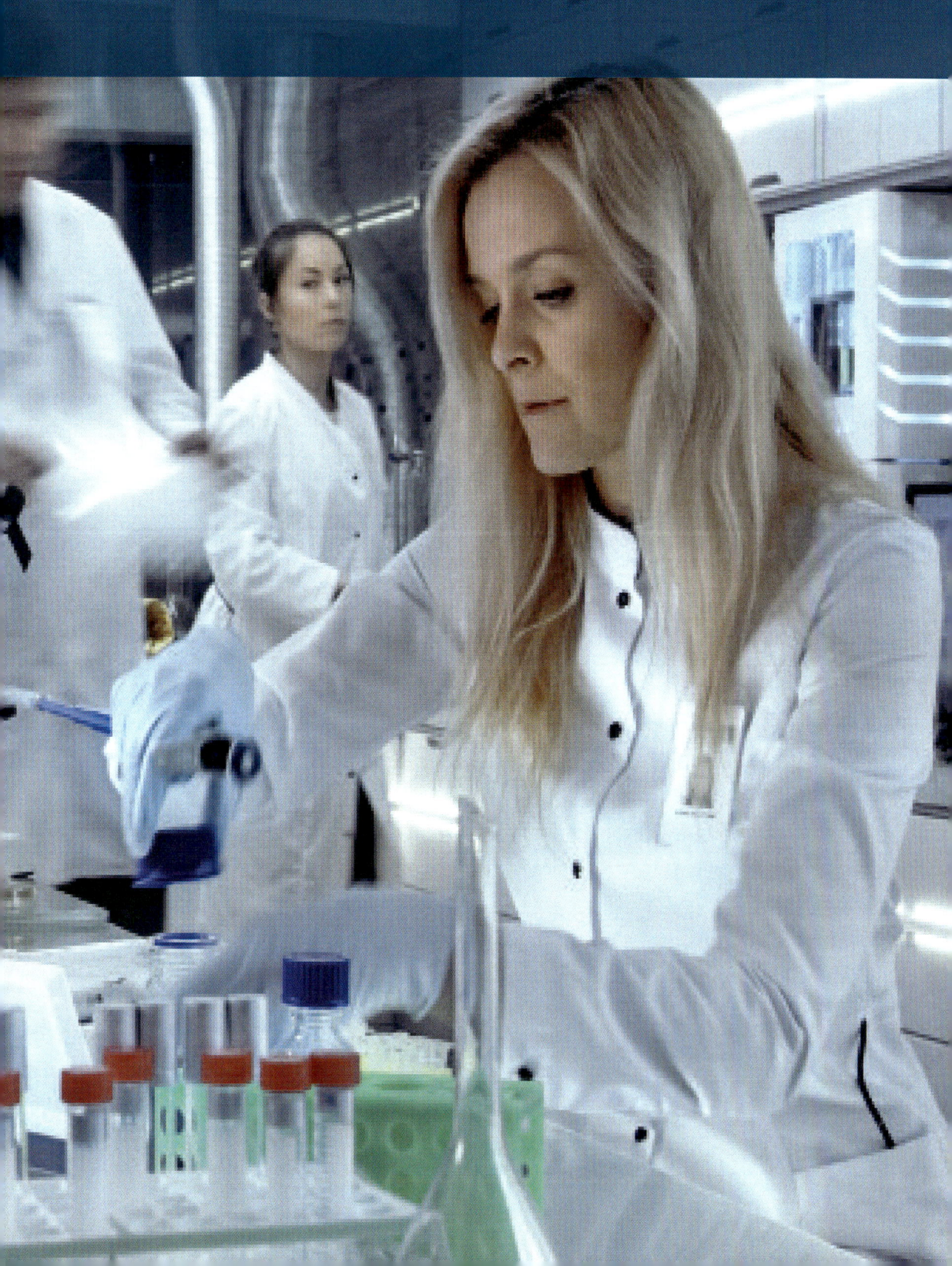

> **"There are no shortcuts to any place worth going."**
>
> **- Beverly Sills**

Following the completion of these exercises, you will be able to:

1. Demonstrate competency in managing critical clinical work processes in long-term care nursing practices, including:
    a. Laboratory processes
    b. Pharmacy processes
    c. Oxygen delivery processes
    d. Transportation processes

2. Evaluate the long-term care nurse's role in managing and coordinating these clinical work processes.

Review Chapter 11 of the training manual, "Navigating Long Term Care: A Practical Approach for Nurses" and then attempt the following questions:

📖 Exercise 1

Describe how you would process a lab order.

_____
_____
_____
_____
_____
_____
_____
_____
_____
_____
_____
_____
_____

Exercise 2

Give a detailed description of how you would process an order for a new medication. Follow your facility's policy, as applicable.

Exercise 3

Describe how you would process and manage a clinician's order for a specialist consult requiring medical transportation services to send a resident for the appointment.

Exercise 4

Give a detailed description of how to process a clinician's order for a STAT chest X-ray.

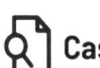

_____

_____

_____

_____

_____

_____

_____

_____

_____

_____

_____

_____

Case Study Review #1

Read the case study below and answer the following questions:

Ms. Hildegard Campbell, who loves to be called "Hilde," is an 87-year-old resident at Akwaaba Skilled Nursing Center. Ms. Campbell woke up one morning complaining of shortness of breath, a productive cough, and refusing all her ADLs. She also refused to eat her breakfast or get out of bed. The nurse was notified about the sudden change in her behavior, and she was assessed, and the findings were recorded in her medical records. The nurse also reviewed the resident's chart to obtain more insights into the resident's condition. See the results below.

Chart Review

Medical History	Medical History	Medication List

Diagnosis:
  o Diabetes Mellitus Type 2
  o Major depressive disorder
  o Hypertension
  o Hyperlipidemia
  o Osteoarthritis
  o Chronic pain
• Advanced Directives: Full code
	• Blood pressure 140/88
	• Pulse 99 +2 regular
	• Respiratory rate 28
	• Temperature 101.6°F
	• SaO2 88% on RA
	• Pain 5/10 to lower back
	• Rapid COVID-19 test -ve
	• Lung sounds with crackles bilat
	• BSx4 quad, normoactive
		• Metformin 500mg PO BID
		• Lisinopril 20mg PO daily
		• Fingerstick three times daily with meals
		• Atorvastatin 20mg at HS
		• Multivitamin 1 tab PO daily
		• Acetaminophen ES 1000mg PO BID

a. Based on her chief complaint and assessment findings, formulate an SBAR to communicate Hilde's change in condition to the covering clinician.

_____

_____

_____

_____

_____

_____

_____

_____

_____

_____

_____

_____

The clinician was notified about the change in condition and gave the following verbal orders:
- Obtain complete blood count (CBC) in am
- Obtain basic metabolic panel (BMP) in am
- Chest X-Ray Stat
- Start resident on oxygen 2L via NC to maintain SaO2>90%

Exercise 5

Complete the work process activities listed below:
- Transcribe the verbal order to the resident's EHR.
- Process the lab and radiology orders as ordered.

At 12:30 pm, the resident's lab and radiology reports were faxed to the unit and were as follows:

CBC Results

Component	Your Value	Standard Range	Flag
WBC	11.2 10*3/uL	4.3-10.8 10*3/uL	H
RBC	4.67 10*6/uL	3.80-5.10 10*6/uL	
Hemoglobin	12.5 g/dL	11.7-15.5 g/dL	
Hematocrit	42.9 %	35.0-46.0 %	
MCV	91.7 fL	80.0-100.0 fL	
MCH	30.9 pg	27.0-34.0 pg	
MCHC	33.7 g/dL	29.0-36.0 g/dL	
RDW	13.8 %	11.0-15.0 %	
Platelets	289 10*3/uL	140-440 10*3/uL	

BMP Results

Component	Your Value	Standard Range	Flag
Sodium	142 mmol/L	136-145 mmol/L	
Potassium	3.8 mmol/L	3.5-5.3 mmol/L	
Chloride	106 mmol/L	97-110 mmol/L	
Carbon Dioxide	25 mmol/L	24-32 mmol/L	
Anion Gap	6	5-15	
Glucose	300 mg/dL	70-99 mg/dL	H
BUN	18 mg/dL	7-23 mg/dL	
Creatinine	0.95 mg/dL	0.5-1.20 mg/dL	
eGFR	>60	>60	

Radiology Report Study Result

FINDINGS AND IMPRESSIONS:
A small area of opacity in the right lower lobe is likely related to developing consolidation or atelectasis. The asymmetric haziness of the right lung compared to the left is related to the technique. Cardio-mediastinal silhouette not enlarged. No pulmonary edema. No pleural effusion or pneumothorax. There is no acute osseous abnormality.

The nurse calls the clinician with the updated results and receives the following verbal orders:
- Azithromycin 500mg x 1 then, 250mg Po daily x 4 days
- Lactobacillus Acidophilus 1 cap PO daily while on antibiotics

Exercise 6

Transcribe the verbal orders to the resident's health record(s) (clinician order forms and MAR/e-MAR), then outline how you will communicate the new orders to the pharmacy.

Day 2 of Treatment
Ms. Hilde continues her antibiotic treatment. However, she is noted have to increased congestion and shortness of breath. Vital signs are BP 128/67, P 113, T 100.6°F RR 30, SaO2 85% on 2L O2 via NC. The NP was notified, and an order was given to transfer the resident to the ER for further evaluation.

Exercise 7

Before the clinician was called, what immediate intervention could the nurse have done considering the resident's oxygenation status? Give a rationale.

📘 Exercise 8

Process the verbal order into the resident's medical records and arrange transportation to the ER. Document your processes below in a nurse's note.

📘 Exercise 9

Assume you are the manager of your unit; how would you coordinate and manage clinical work processes such as pharmacy, laboratory, oxygen, and transportation services?

Self-Reflective Exercise

Stop for a few minutes and reflect by asking yourself these questions.

1. How competent am I at transcribing clinician orders?
2. How competent am I at processing orders to the lab?
3. How competent am I at processing orders at the pharmacy?
4. How competent am I at booking transportation?
5. Do I hesitate to ask for help from my peers? Why?
6. Do I readily offer to help peers with processing orders?
7. How can I be more helpful to my peers and foster a team spirit?

My Journal

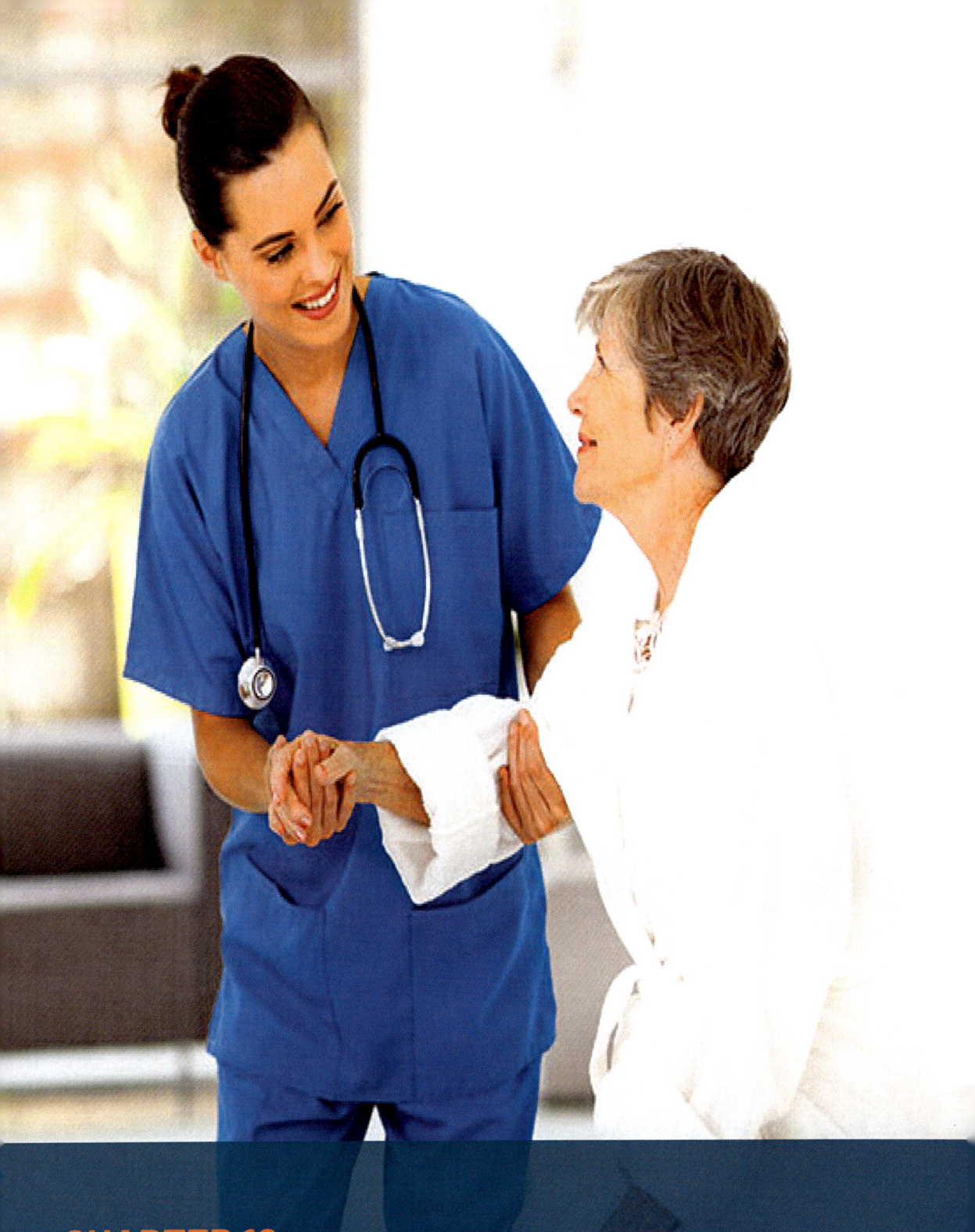

CHAPTER 12:
RESIDENT CARE DELIVERY PROCESS

> "It's not how much you do, but how much love you put into the doing."
>
> **- Mother Teresa**

Following the completion of these exercises, you will be able to:
1. Demonstrate competency in the resident admission process.
2. Demonstrate competency in the resident care planning process.
3. Demonstrate competency in an acute transfer process in a long-term care facility.
4. Understand the role of the nurse in discharge planning.

Review Chapter 12 of the training manual, "Navigating Long Term Care: A Practical Approach for Nurses", and then attempt the following exercises:

Admission Process

Figure 1: A sample hospital discharge summary.

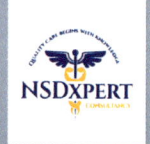

NSDXPERT

NSD Hospital

Kojo Abbeyquaye, MD Physician   H&P   Date of Service: 1/6/2023   2:32pm

HISTORY AND PHYSICAL

Mary A Banson; 6/19/1945, 78-year-old female

CHIEF COMPLAINT:
Worsening confusion

HISTORY OF PRESENT ILLNESS

This is an 88-year-old female with a history of dementia, urinary retention with a chronic Foley catheter, and hypertension who presented to the ER at NSD Hospital for aggressive behaviors at home. The patient removed her Foley catheter last night and did not let a visiting nurse place another Foley catheter.

According to the patient's daughter, the patient lives alone but has visiting nurses and 24x7 home care providers. The patient reportedly has been getting increasingly agitated and combative with care towards staff. The patient's primary care doctor was contacted and recommended sending the patient to the ER for further evaluation and Foley catheter placement. In addition, the patient has a history of multiple urinary tract infections in the past, requiring hospitalization.

In the ER, she was agitated and combative with staff. ER, physicians could not examine her appropriately. They were able to obtain blood work and urine analysis. The blood work looks okay, but the urine analysis is abnormal and positive for urinary tract infection. The patient was given a dose of Cefepime® based on the sensitivities of urine culture. The patient had a history of ESBL in the past. Medical admission is requested due to behavioral disturbances likely exacerbated by a urinary tract infection.

No history of fever, chills, nausea, vomiting, constipation, or diarrhea. No history of headache, loss of consciousness, or seizure activity. She is moving all extremities during my evaluation in the ER. She is unable to follow any commands.

PHYSICAL EXAM:
General: confused, unable to follow directions appropriately, no acute distress
HEENT: normocephalic, atraumatic, moist oral mucosa.
Lymphatic: no lymphadenopathy
Respiratory: fair air entry bilaterally, no wheezes, no rhonchi
Cardiovascular: S1, and S2 are present. No rubs or gallops. Regular rate and rhythm
GI: Soft, non-tender, no guarding, no rigidity, normal bowel sounds.
Genitourinary: no CVA tenderness
Neuro: awake, alert, confused, moving all extremities
Extremities: warm, no cyanosis, no clubbing, pulses present
Skin: warm and dry

ASSESSMENT AND PLAN
1. Acute encephalopathy due to urinary tract infection
    - The patient started on cefepime 1 g IV every 8 hours.
    - Follow urine cultures and sensitivities.
2. Dementia with behavioral disturbances
    - Continue supportive care with fall and aspiration precautions.
3. GERD
    - Continue Pepcid.

Enoxaparin Sodium (Lovenox®) subcutaneous for DVT prophylaxis
Code status confirmed DNR/DNI

The patient's daughter is the healthcare proxy, and treatment has been discussed with her, and she agrees.

Based on the history, comorbidities, severity of signs and symptoms, current medical needs, and risk of an adverse event, I expect this patient's care to require 2 overnights in the hospital.

PRINCIPAL PROBLEM:
Acute metabolic encephalopathy
Active Problems:
Hypertension
Gastroesophageal reflux disease (GERD)
History of Stroke
Urinary Retention

Current Hospital Administered Medications

Medication	Dose	Route	Frequency	Provider
Acetaminophen tablet 650 mg	650mg	Oral	Q6h PRN	Kojo Abbeyquaye, MD
Aripiprazole tablet 2 mg	2mg	Oral	daily	Kojo Abbeyquaye, MD
Cefepime 1 g in 0.9% NaCl 100 ml	1g	Intravenous	3x daily	Kojo Abbeyquaye, MD
Docusate Sodium capsule 100 mg	100mg	Oral	2x daily	Kojo Abbeyquaye, MD
Enoxaparin subcutaneous injection 40 mg	40mg	Subcutaneous	daily	Kojo Abbeyquaye, MD
Famotidine tablet 20 mg Start on 1/6/2023	20mg	Oral	Daily	Kojo Abbeyquaye, MD
Lactobacillus acidophilus- L bulgaricus 1 tablet	1 tab	Oral	2x daily	Kojo Abbeyquaye, MD
Mirtazapine tablet 15 mg	15mg	Oral	Nightly	Kojo Abbeyquaye, MD
Senna tablet 17.2 mg	17.2 mg	Oral	Nightly	Kojo Abbeyquaye, MD
Trazodone tablet 50 mg	50mg	Oral	Nightly PRN	Kojo Abbeyquaye, MD
Venlafaxine XR capsule 150 mg Start on 1/6/2023	150mg	Oral	Daily with breakfast	Kojo Abbeyquaye, MD

Current Outpatient Medications

Lisinopril 5 mg tablet take   1 tablet by mouth daily   dispense 30 tablets   0 Refill
Omeprazole 20 mg capsule   take 20mg by mouth daily   0 refill
Pravastatin 10 mg tablet   take 10mg by mouth daily   0 refill
Venlafaxine 75 mg   take 225 mg by mouth daily   0 refill
Verapamil 120 mg tablet   take 1 tablet 120mg by mouth every 8 hours
                                                                                                    Dispense 90 tablets   0 refill

REVIEW OF SYSTEMS
Other systems were reviewed, and they were negative.

FAMILY HISTORY

Problem	Relation
Diabetes	Sister
Tuberculosis	Mother
Hypertension	Mother
Coronary Artery disease (CAD)	Mother, Father

SOCIAL HISTORY

Marital status	Widowed
Number of Children	4
Years of education	not on file
Highest education level	College

Occupational history
Registered nurse

Tobacco use	Never smoker
Alcohol use	Not in the last 40+ years
Drug use	never

PAST MEDICAL HISTORY

Chronic lower back
Breast cancer s/p R mastectomy
Depression with anxiety
Essential hypertension
Fatty Liver
Frequent falls at home
History of stroke
Hyperlipidemia
Osteoporosis
Peripheral vascular disease
Recurrent UTI

ALLERGIES

Aspirin
Latex
Codeine

Prior to Admission Medications

Lisinopril 5 mg –	take 5mg by mouth daily	Joe Doe MD
Omeprazole 20 mg –	take 20mg by mouth daily	Joe Doe MD
Pravastatin 10 mg –	take 10 mg by mouth daily	Joe Doe MD
Effexor 75mg tablet –	take 225mg by mouth daily	Joe Doe MD
Verapamil 120mg tab –	Take 1 tab (120mg) by mouth every 8 hours	Joe Doe MD

Recent lab results (from the past 24 hours)

Rapid COVID-19 for surveillance collected 1/6/2023 at 3:00pm
Result
Rapid SARS CoV-2   Negative

CBC with Diff

Component	Value	Ref Range	Flag
WBC	11.2 10*3/uL	4.3 - 10.8 10*3/uL	H
RBC	4.67 10*6/uL	3.80 - 5.10 10*6/uL	
Hemoglobin	12.5 g/dL	11.7 - 15.5 g/dL	
Hematocrit	42.9 %	35.0 - 46.0 %	
MCV	91.7 fL	80.0 - 100.0 fL	
MCH	30.9 pg	27.0 - 34.0 pg	
MCHC	33.7 g/dL	29.0 - 36.0 g/dL	
RDW	13.8 %	11.0 - 15.0 %	
Platelets	479 10*3/uL	140 - 440 10*3/uL	H
MPV	7.6	7.6 -11.6 fL	
Neutrophils	58.1	%	
Lymphocyte	32.2	%	
Monocyte	6.6	%	
Eosinophil	2.1	%	
Basophil	1.0	%	

CMP- Comprehensive Panel   collected 1/6/23 at 6:44 pm

Component	Value	Ref Range	
NA	141	136 – 145 mmol/L	
K	4.0	3.5 -5.3 mmol/L	
Cl	108	97-110 mmol/L	
CO2	25	24-32 mmol/L	
Anion Gap	8	5-15	
Glucose	112	70-99 mg/dL	H
Creatinine	0.68	0.5-1.20 mg/dL	
Total protein	7.3	6.0-8.0 g/dL	
Albumin	3.8	3.5-5.0 g/dL	
Bilirubin, total	0.4	0.3-1.2 mg/dL	
Alkaline phosphatase	74	30-115 U/L	
AST	24	10-40 U/L	
ALT	18	10-40 U/L	
BUN	25	7-23	H

UA C & S - Urinalysis and culture collected 1/6/23 at 7.05 pm.

Component	Value	Ref range	
Color Urine	yellow	Yellow	
Clarity Urine	cloudy	Clear	A
Protein, Urine	positive	Negative	A
Glucose Urine	negative	Negative	
Ketones Urine	trace	Negative	A
Blood Urine	moderate	Negative	A
Nitrite Urine	Positive	Negative	A
Leukocyte esterase, Urine large	Negative		A
Bacteria, Urine	4+	None	A

Culture pending

I have reviewed the laboratory results.
I have personally reviewed and summarized old records and previous discharge summaries.

Electronically signed by Kojo Abbeyquaye, MD 1/9/2023   12:00 p.m.

DISCHARGE PLAN
You were admitted because of your confusion and aggressive behavior. Your symptoms are likely due to the acute onset of a urinary tract infection. We will transfer to a skilled nursing facility to complete IV antibiotic therapy and skilled rehabilitation for general weakness.

DISCHARGE INSTRUCTIONS
Some of your medications have changed during your visit.
Please refer to your medication reconciliation sheet for a complete list of your discharge medications.

Appointments
Follow up with a urologist for a recurrent UTI.
Psychiatric consultation is recommended.

General Instructions
Diet as tolerated.
Transportation is to be arranged by case management.

Your Complete Medication list as of 1/9/2023

Acetaminophen	650 mg by mouth every 6 hours as needed.
Aripiprazole	2 mg by mouth daily
Cefepime	1 g in 0.9% NaCl 100mg Intravenously daily x 4 more doses
Docusate Sodium	100mg by mouth twice daily
Famotidine	20 mg by mouth daily

Lactobacillus acidophilus	1 tablet by mouth twice daily
Mirtazapine	15mg by mouth daily at night
Senna	17.2 mg by mouth daily
Trazodone	50mg by mouth at bedtime as needed
Venlafaxine XR	150mg by mouth daily with breakfast

Exercise 1

As the nurse assigned to Ms. Mary Banson on the Geri Psych unit, you are asked to admit her to RM 204. Outline what you will do first when she arrives at the nursing unit. *(Refer to the sample hospital discharge and chapter 12 of your training manual to complete this exercise)*

_____
_____
_____
_____
_____
_____
_____
_____
_____
_____
_____

Exercise 2

Use the admission checklist in Appendix A of your training manual as a guide to admitting Ms. Banson to the unit. In addition, your admission should include the following processes:

- Obtaining all relevant legal consents. (Follow your facility policy)
- Admission intake assessment (Comprehensive)
- Risk Assessment
- Medication reconciliation process
- Physician order processes- (Clinician order verification, transcription, and processing to appropriate departments)
- Admission care planning process (Develop at least five initial care plans for Ms. Banson)
  (You may use the training site of your facility's EHR where applicable)

Exercise 3

Write a detailed admission nursing note.

___

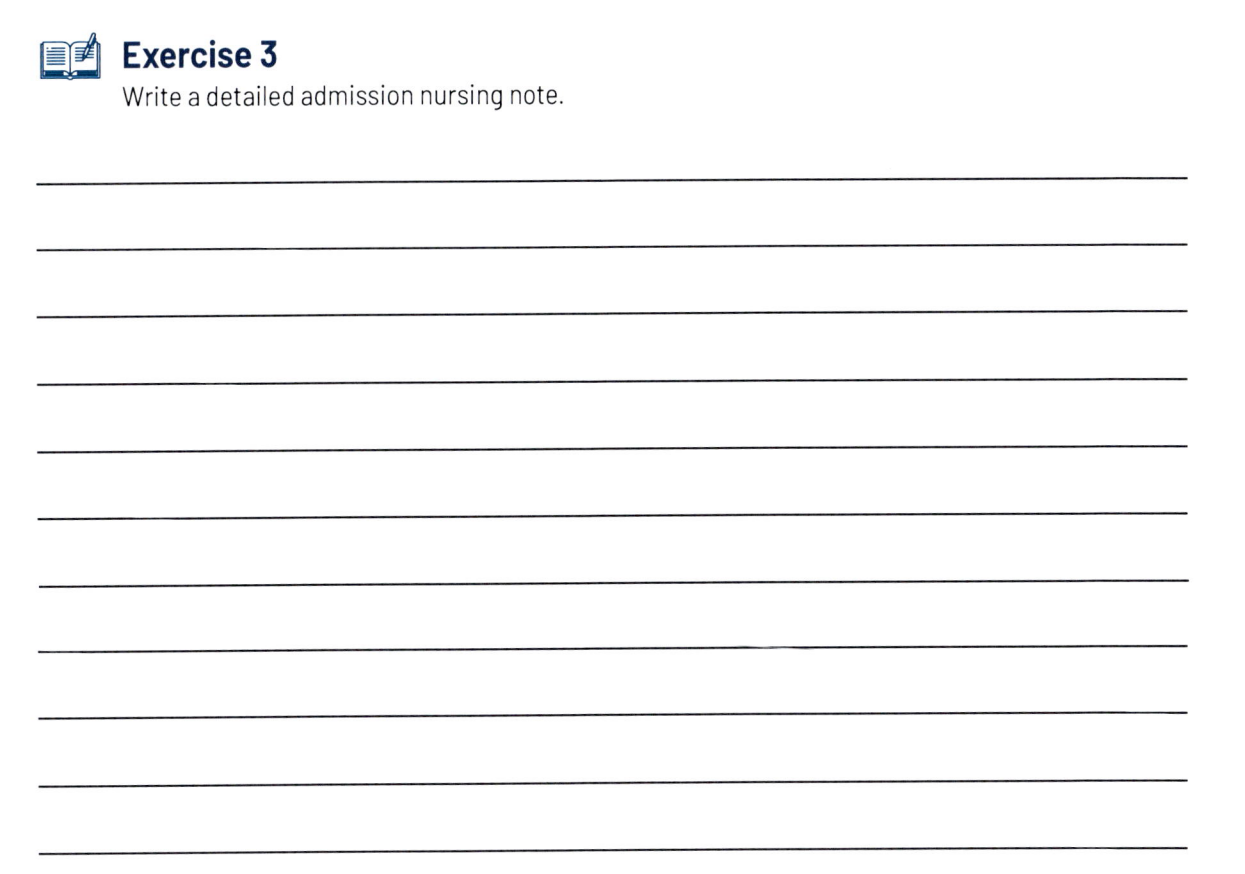

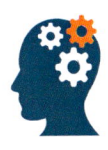

Clinical Skills Competency

- Blood pressure measurement
  - » Manual
  - » Electronic
- Radial and apical pulse taking
- Respiration
- Temperature measurement
  - » Oral
  - » Tympanic
  - » Rectal
  - » Axilla
- Weighing a resident
  - » Resident in a wheelchair
- Obtaining resident height
  - » Standing
  - » Lying

- Body systems assessment (head-to-toe)
  - » Neurological assessment
  - » Cardiovascular system assessment
  - » Respiratory system assessment
  - » Gastrointestinal system assessment
  - » Genitourinary system assessment
  - » Musculoskeletal system assessment

Exercise 4

Five days after admitting Ms. Banson, her daughter visits and is unhappy with the care her mother is receiving at the facility. She wants her discharged immediately despite receiving medical advice from the clinician. As the nurse assigned to the resident, what should you do to ensure a safe "AMA" discharge? (You may refer to your facility's policy)

Case Study Review #1

Review the case scenario about Ms. Buckman on page 193 of your training manual and complete the activity below.

a. Transcribe the clinician's verbal order to the resident's health records.
b. Gather and complete all required legal and regulatory documents needed to transfer Ms. Buckman to the ER (Refer to chapter 12 of your training manual for guidance)
c. Gather and complete all clinical documents needed to transfer Ms. Buckman. Do not forget to complete an SBAR! (Refer to the training manual)
d. Write an acute transfer nursing note for Ms. Buckman.

Discharge Planning

📖 Exercise 5

Participate in a discharge planning meeting and evaluate the process and the role of the nurse within the process. Write your findings below.

Exercise 6

A nurse was asked to complete pages 1 and 2 of the discharge summary for a resident who was scheduled to be discharged home. What information would they include in the:

a. Page 1?

b. Page 2?

Exercise 7
For Registered Nurses Only

Describe the process of death pronouncement by a registered nurse in a skilled nursing facility.

Self-Reflective Exercise

Stop for a few minutes and reflect by asking yourself these questions.

1. What is my attitude when I am assigned to complete an admission?
2. How confident am I in handling resident admissions?
3. What process of the admission process may keep me up at night?
4. How confident am I in completing a head-to-toe assessment?
5. How competent am I in handling an acute resident transfer?
6. How competent am I at completing a discharge summary?
7. Do I assist my peers in completing admissions even if it is not assigned to me?
8. Do I readily ask for help with admissions from peers?
9. How can I be more helpful to my peers and foster a team spirit?
10. How confident am I in completing a care plan?
11. What can I do to improve my competency in completing a resident admission?

My Journal

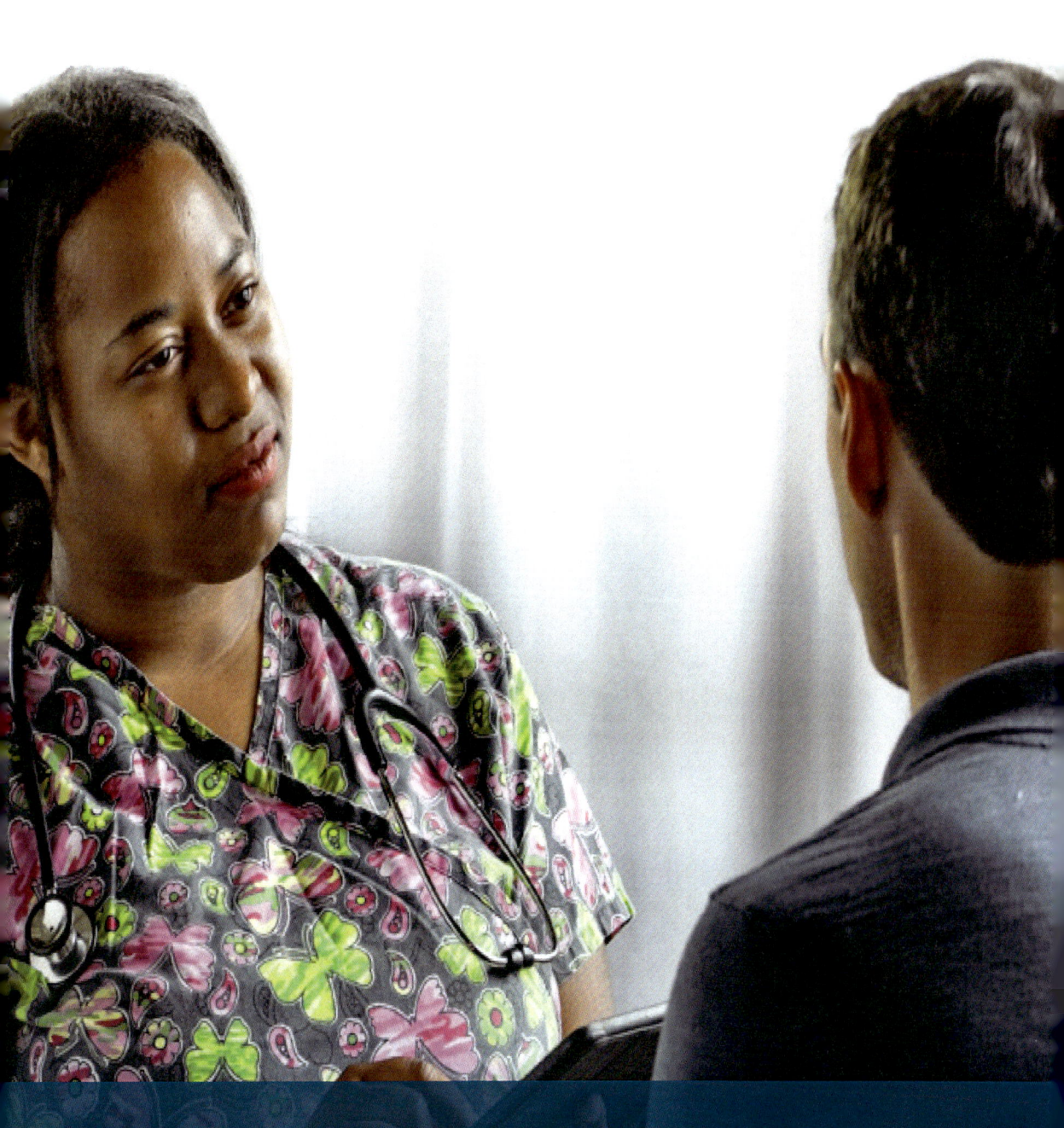

CHAPTER 13:

NURSING ASSESSMENTS

Following the completion of these exercises, you will be able to:
1. Describe common assessment instruments used in long-term care settings.
2. Analyze assessment findings and intervene to ensure resident safety.
3. Demonstrate competency in completing common assessment instruments used in long-term care settings.
4. Evaluate the nurse's role in residents' assessments.

📖 Exercise 1

At Akwaaba Skilled Nursing and Rehabilitation Center, assessments are expected to follow the schedule outlined on **page 208** of the training manual. For example, the nurse should complete the following evaluations for newly admitted residents to establish their baseline status and meet their care needs:

- Comprehensive Resident Admission Assessment
- Health and physical
- Elopement Risk
- Bed Rail Evaluation
- Fall Risk
- Smoking Risk
- Pressure Injury Risk
- Cognitive Status
- Bowel and Bladder
- Educational Need
- Functional Ability (Section GG of MDS)
- AIMS
- Nutritional Assessment
- Trauma Assessment
- Safe Use of Mechanical Lift

a. Ms. Mary Banson, in the previous chapter, was admitted to the Geri psych unit. As the nurse tasked to complete her admission, complete a fall risk assessment using the Briggs fall risk **assessment (See Appendix E of your training manual)**

b. Interpret and analyze your fall assessment finding(s). (Refer to **Chapter 13** of your training manual)

c. Describe how your findings may influence the plan of care for Ms. Banson.

d. On admission, Ms. Banson's Norton Plus Pressure Ulcer score was 8. Analyze her risk for pressure injury and then develop a plan to educate the Certified Nurse Assistants (CNAs) working on the unit. Your plan must include methods of evaluating their understanding of Ms. Banson's pressure injury risks.

Exercise 2

What is the Abnormal Involuntary Movement Scale (AIMS), and why do we need the AIMS assessment to be completed for only specific residents?

Exercise 3

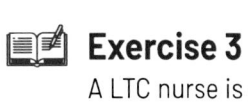

A LTC nurse is completing the monthly nursing summary for Ms. Chun Wong. During the review of Ms. Wong's ADL flow sheets, they notice that the CNAs have documented that she has had bladder incontinence more than 20 times in the month. The nurse confirms that the finding is a change from the previous month. Outline in detail what the nurse should do.

Group Activity #1

Identify a resident at your facility who is at risk for bladder or bowel incontinence. Complete a bladder or bowel evaluation and determine if they are candidates for retraining.

_____
_____
_____
_____
_____
_____
_____
_____
_____
_____
_____
_____
_____

Exercise 4

Describe what the nurse would do when asked to initiate a bladder or bowel retraining for a resident.

_____
_____
_____
_____
_____
_____
_____
_____
_____

Exercise 5

During a care plan meeting for Mr. Brew, the certified nurse assistant indicated that Mr. Brew's hands had been shaking a lot, and there had been a few times in recent weeks when he had dropped his cigarette. The certified nurse aide expressed concern for his safety during smoking to the team. Describe what the nurse should do in order of priority.

Exercise 6

The nurse is admitting a new resident to the subacute unit. The resident states, "I would like to keep my inhaler at my bedside and administer it myself." What should the nurse do?

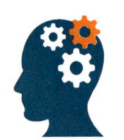

Clinical Skills Competency

The nurse should demonstrate competency in completing these assessment tools as part of training.
- Fall Risk Assessment
- Brief Interview for Mental Status (BIMS)
- Montreal Cognitive Assessment (MOCA)
- Braden Scale
- Norton Scale
- Section GG of Minimum Data Set
- Elopement Risk Assessment
- Smoking Risk Assessment
- Abnormal Involuntary Movement Scale (AIMS)
- Bed Rail Assessment Tool
- Bowel and Bladder Continence Assessment
- 3-Day Bowel and Bladder Diary

Self-Reflective Exercise

Stop for a few minutes and reflect by asking yourself these questions.

1. Do I take time to review a resident's medical record when completing an assessment?
2. How readily do I complete resident assessments?
3. Do I feel competent in completing resident assessments?
4. What is my attitude when asked to complete a resident assessment?
5. How vital is a resident assessment to me?

My Journal

CHAPTER 14:
INCIDENT REPORTING PROCESSES

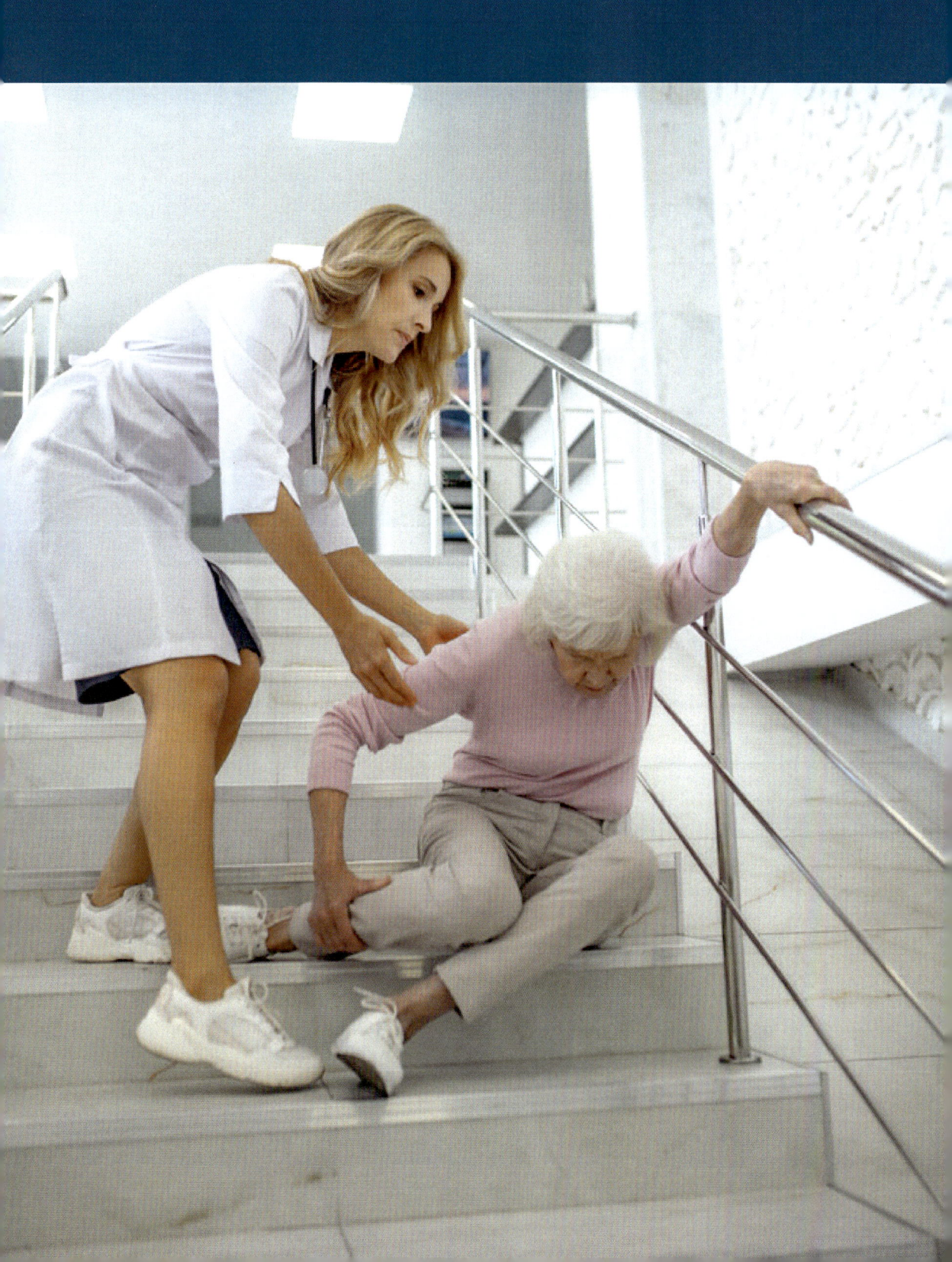

> *"Every incident is a notice that something is wrong with men, methods, or material – investigate – then act."*
>
> **- Unknown Author**

Following the completion of these exercises, you will be able to:

1. Explain incident reporting and investigation processes of common incidents in long-term care facilities.
2. Demonstrate competence in reporting and investigating incidents in long-term care settings.
3. Apply the nursing process in incident reporting and investigation.
4. Interpret the nurse's role in Quality Assurance and Performance Improvement (QAPI) processes.

Review Chapter 14 of the training manual, *"Navigating Long Term Care: A Practical Approach for Nurses"*, and then attempt the following exercises:

Fall Incidents

Case Study Review #1

Refer to the case study on page 226 of the training manual and answer the questions below.

a. What should Nurse Brown do next?

_____
_____
_____
_____
_____
_____
_____
_____
_____
_____
_____
_____
_____
_____
_____

b. Outline a task plan for Nurse Brown based on the facility's policies and procedures.

c. Complete a comprehensive fall incident report. (Follow your facility policy)

Group Activity #1

As part of the incident reporting process, witness statements were obtained from staff working on the units, such as:

- "I was feeding another resident and did not witness the fall."
- "I was on break. I do not know what happened."
- "I did not have the resident."
- "I do not know what happened."
- "I heard a big sound and listened to the resident calling for help. I went in and saw her on the floor and called the nurse. I do not know what happened."

Analyze and critique these statements and indicate whether further information may have been helpful to the investigation.

📖 Exercise 1

Practice writing a fall witness statement for the incident described in the case scenario.

📖 Exercise 2

Write a fall incident note for the case scenario presented.

New Pressure Injury Incident

Case Study Review #2

Refer to the case study on page 228 of your training manual and answer the following questions:

a. Outline the nurse's tasks in the order of priority in the initial investigation and reporting of this incident.

b. What should the nurse do in assessing the situation?

c. If you were the nurse, what questions would you ask regarding this incident?

d. Describe in detail the process of handling a new pressure incident in your facility.

e. List a few interventions you would implement to manage the wound on Mr. Arnold's buttock.

Burn Incidents

Case Study Review #3

Refer to the case study on page 230 and answer the following questions:

a. Using the nursing process as a guide, outline how to investigate and handle this incident step by step.

___

b. Review Chapter 14 of the training manual and outline a task plan to handle burn incidents. (You may use your facility's policy and procedures).

___

c. Discuss some interventions that could be implemented to prevent a future occurrence and note the key points discussed. **(Group activity)**

_____

_____

_____

_____

_____

_____

_____

_____

_____

_____

d. Write an incident note for this case. **(Trainees should discuss and critique each other's notes)**

_____

_____

_____

_____

_____

_____

_____

_____

_____

Abuse/Neglect/ Misappropriation

Case Study Review #4

The Director of Nursing received a call from Ms. Benedicta Adams, a family member, who stated that she had just received a bill on her mother's credit card and was worried since her mother, Mary Guy, could not have been using the card. An investigation was initiated immediately, and an abuse report was filed with the local police department and the Department of Public Health. Ms. Mary Guy is an 86-year-old who is pleasantly confused at baseline due to dementia and loves to carry her favorite purse everywhere. According to the staff, the credit card is usually kept in her purse but was noted as missing. Staff was interviewed, but they denied knowledge of the incident. About a week later, a staff member was arrested at the facility for using the card at multiple department stores located about 40 miles from the facility.

A. What lessons can be learned from this case?

B. What could the facility have done to prevent this incident?

C. What can you do as a long-term care nurse to prevent such incidents at your facility?

Unexpected Death Incident

Case Study Review #5

Review the case study on page 235 of the training manual and answer the following questions:

a.   What should Nurse Lucky do in the scenario described?

b.   Outline a task plan that would help Nurse Lucky handle the situation.

c. An internal review of the emergency response by staff was found to be suboptimal, warranting training and competency in CPR and emergency response. As a group, develop a lesson plan incorporating CPR and AED competency.

Group Activity #2

Identify residents that have high-risk scores on their elopement assessment and, as a group, develop an elopement alert book for your unit. Be creative!

Quality Assurance and Performance Improvement (QAPI) Processes

Exercise 3

Attend a QAPI meeting at your facility and write about your experience.

Exercise 4

Identify an issue(s) at your facility that you could bring to the QAPI team.

___

Exercise 5

Select any one of the issues presented and form a mock QAPI team with your peers to develop a plan that could be implemented to fix the issue. Your project must be creative and include a plan to educate staff.

___

Self-Reflective Exercise

Stop for a few minutes and reflect by asking yourself these questions.

1. Do I feel competent in completing an incident report?
2. What is my attitude toward completing an incident report?
3. How do I feel when wrongly accused of resident abuse/neglect/misappropriation?
4. How do I feel when asked to go home based on an allegation of abuse?
5. Am I doing enough to keep vulnerable residents safe?
6. What do I do for my residents when no one is looking?
7. Do I take time to supervise residents during mealtime?
8. Do I question or report suboptimal resident care when I see it?
9. What can I do to minimize falls at my facility?
10. Do I sleep on the job instead of rounding on my residents at night?

My Journal